Viral Diseases of the Central Nervous System

Edited by

L. S. ILLIS
Consultant Neurologist, Wessex Neurological Centre,
Southampton General Hospital; Clinical Senior Lecturer,
University of Southampton Medical School

with a foreword by

D. CARLETON GAJDUSEK
Chief of the Laboratory of Slow, Latent and Temperate
Virus Infections, National Institutes of Health, USA

LONDON ✤ BAILLIÈRE TINDALL

BAILLIÈRE TINDALL
7 & 8 Henrietta Street, London WC2E 8QE

Cassell & Collier Macmillan Publishers Ltd., London
35 Red Lion Square, London WC1R 4SG
Sydney, Auckland, Toronto, Johannesburg

The Macmillan Publishing Company Inc.
New York

First published 1975

ISBN 0 7020 0575 4

Printed in Great Britain by R. & R. Clark Ltd., Edinburgh

Contributors

J. HUME ADAMS MBChB, PhD, FRCPath, MRCP (Glasg)
Professor of Neuropathology, Institute of Neuropathological Sciences, Southern General Hospital, Glasgow

JUNE D. ALMEIDA DSc
Wellcome Research Laboratories, Beckenham, Kent

W. A. COBB FRCP
Consultant Clinical Neurophysiologist, National Hospital for Nervous Diseases, Queen Square, London

A. D. DAYAN MD, MRCP, MRCPath
Wellcome Research Laboratories, Beckenham, Kent

G. W. A. DICK MD, DSc, FRCP, FRCPath
Assistant Director, British Postgraduate Medical Federation

E. J. FIELD MD, MS, PhD, FRCP
Professor of Experimental Neuropathology, University of Newcastle, Newcastle General Hospital, Newcastle upon Tyne

J. V. T. GOSTLING MA, MB, BChir, FRCPath
Consultant Virologist, Public Health Labratory, Portsmouth

L. S. ILLIS   MD, BSc, FRCP
Consultant Neurologist, Wessex Neurological Centre; Clinical Senior Lecturer, University of Southampton Medical School, Southampton

M. LONGSON   MD, BSc
Consultant Virologist, North Manchester Regional Virus Laboratory, Manchester Royal Infirmary

W. B. MATTHEWS   DM, FRCP
Professor of Clinical Neurology, University of Oxford

D. R. OPPENHEIMER   DM
Honorary Consultant Neuropathologist, Radcliffe Infirmary, Oxford

H. E. WEBB   DM, FRCP
Consultant Neurologist and Senior Lecturer in Medicine, St Thomas's Hospital Medical School, London

I. ZLOTNIK   PhD, BVSc, MRCVS
Head of Experimental Pathology, Microbiological Research Establishment, Porton Down, Salisbury, Wiltshire.

Foreword

It is good to have this new summary of virus diseases of the central nervous system, written exclusively by our colleagues in the United Kingdom, from where so much of the interest in viruses as the cause of subacute and chronic infections has originated. I am especially pleased to have this British summary of slow, latent and temperate virus infections in the section on transmissible and degenerative diseases of the nervous system. It is based largely on the group of transmissible infections we have defined as the subacute spongiform virus encephalopathies, which include two diseases of man, kuru and transmissible virus dementia, and two diseases of animals, scrapie of sheep and goats and transmissible mink encephalopathy (TME). The careful distinction we have been forced to make between the infections caused by unconventional viruses, i.e. the agents of the subacute spongiform virus encephalopathies (SSVE), and those caused by conventional viruses—wherein the slowness of the infection is regulated by an abnormal or immature immunological state in the host (as in progressive multifocal leuco-encephalopathy) or by other factors which may result in defective virus replication or asynchronous production of virus subunits and incomplete or absent assembly of fully infectious virions (as in subacute sclerosing panencephalitis)—is happily preserved.

I agree with the authors who wisely avoid controversy, until further information is available, as to just which dementia syndromes of the spongiform group, including those usually called Creutzfeldt–Jakob disease (CJD), are transmissible virus dementias. Already the range of dementias of man transmitted as SSVE to subhuman primates extends beyond the syndrome called CJD and embraces diseases associated with a variety of other neuropathological reactions, such as the variable presence of amyloid plaques, neurofibrillary tangles, granulovacuolar degeneration, Pick's cells, vascular lesions and cellular inclusions. Many pathologists would differ with the claim that changes caused by SSVE viruses are indistinguishable from those of acute virus infections in immunosuppressed animals, but the recognition of the dependence of pathogenesis on the immune responsiveness of the host and the discussion of virulence variants of scrapie and their ease of selection are valuable contributions. The well-reasoned and cautious evaluations of the problems surrounding clinical and pathological diagnosis of the presenile dementias, and the possible relationship of the transmissible virus dementias to some cases which may currently be given other diagnoses, are important.

Clinical and laboratory findings in the acute virus diseases of the nervous system, as they are seen in Britain, are expertly reviewed and antiviral chemotherapy is thoroughly discussed.

Speculations invited by the demonstration that a few rare, chronic noninflammatory, sometimes heredofamilial degenerations of the CNS may be of viral aetiology have understandably stimulated the hopes and hypotheses that such an aetiology may underlie other more common idiopathic disorders, such as multiple sclerosis, amyotrohpic lateral sclerosis, Parkinson's disease and parkinsonism–dementia, but substantiation of such constructions has not yet been achieved. Defective or incompletely expressed synthesis of conventional viruses, or even integration of all or part of their genome into the host's genetic material, are possibilities compelling investigation. Whether atypical viruses of the kuru-CJD–scrapie–TME group, now called the SSVEs, are also to be found in other diseases, is a challenging problem, as is the natural history of these infections.

Perhaps the most important result of the elucidation of these unconventional viruses may lie in the newer insights into the molecular basis of pathogenesis which we will possess once the structure of these apparent membrane subunits is fully unravelled. They have opened a new chapter of mammalian microbiology and there are many indications that they may be a new type of virus with very small pieces of genetic information—many of us have rashly and perhaps prematurely conjectured that this may even be borne on macromolecular structures other than purine–pyrimidine chains—linking the pathogenesis of human disease to that of the smallest replicating viruses or virus subunits in bacteria and plants. Already they have brought us to a reconsideration of the interaction of the immune response with virus modification and evolution and disease pathogenesis.

It is at this critical juncture in the investigation of these degenerative diseases that this new summary appears. In due time it will become out of date, and we will welcome the advances that make it so, but in the meantime it will serve admirably its intended function as a much-needed and up-to-date critical review of this emerging field of medicine.

April 1975   D. CARLETON GAJDUSEK

Preface

This book, based on a recent symposium is written for clinicians (including neurologists and paediatricians), neuro-pathologists and virologists. In the past twenty years there has been a considerable change in the understanding and importance of viral encephalitis. For example, certain conditions previously labelled as 'degenerative' diseases of the central nervous system have been shown to have a transmissible, if not a viral origin, and it is clear that virus infection of the central nervous system may possibly play an important, if not causative, role in many diseases, including multiple sclerosis and amyotrophic lateral sclerosis. Furthermore, it has been postulated that subacute viral infections, particularly herpes simplex virus, may result in brain damage leading to temporal lobe epilepsy and even psychotic disorders. Although acute infections and disorders such as the spongiform encephalopathies are apparently quite distinct, there are certain common features of virus encephalitis of acute, subacute, persistent and 'slow' forms, such as the fact that altered host–virus relationships and altered immune state may change characteristic patterns to different forms, as indicated in Dr Zlotnik's paper.

Thus the problem of viral disease of the central nervous system is assuming a greater importance with the recognition of the varied manifestations of the many forms of virus infection and the possible part played by these infections in other neurological conditions. Infections due to a specific virus have been more frequently recognized and diagnosed and specific syndromes have been delineated as, for example, in herpes simplex encephalitis.

More or less over the same period of time, antiviral agents have become available for study and for general use, although until recently encephalitis has been considered untreatable. The march of antiviral chemotherapy in no way parallels the rapid development of antibacterial agents but there is clear indication of progress in antiviral therapy. Together with the extremely important progress in the knowledge of virus disease, due largely to the interaction of morphologists and virologists, as for example in subacute sclerosing leuco-encephalitis and progressive multifocal leuco-encephalopathy, the future is both bright and interesting.

This growth of knowledge of viral encephalitis and increase in interest in the subject led to the Southampton symposium in May 1974. This book is not a record of the proceedings, but the editor has used the symposium as a basis commissioning additional contributions on several important aspects to produce a balanced picture of encephalitis today. The book is divided into two parts but the sub-division is only intended as a guide to the reader and not to suggest any rigid division.

A book of this kind must rely greatly on the writings of others. Every effort has been made to give due acknowledgment and the editor begs forgiveness of any commentator whose work has been inadvertently overlooked.

April 1975   L. S. ILLIS

Acknowledgements

We are grateful to the publishers and authors listed below for their permission to reproduce the following figures. Fig. 1 from D. Williams (1967), *Modern Trends in Neurology*, London: Butterworths. Fig. 2 from A. Upton and J. Gumpert (1970), *Lancet*, i, 650. Fig. 3 from W. A. Cobb (1968), in *Clinical Electroencephalography of Children*, ed. P. Kellaway and I. Petersen, Stockholm: Almqvist & Wiksel. Some tables in Chapter 6 have been reproduced from the *Journal of the Royal College of Physicians* (1972) and from L. S. Illis and J. V. T. Gostling (1972), *Herpes Simplex Encephalitis*, Bristol: Scientechnica. Dr G. M. Zu Rhein kindly provided the specimen for Plate II/1. Plates VII/1 and VII/3 are reproduced by courtesy of Mrs E. Beck, and Plate VII/4 by courtesy of Professor J. Hume Adams. Finally, it is a pleasure to thank Miss Brenda Meyer for many hours of patient secretarial work.

L. S. I.

Contents

PART ONE

Acute and Subacute Encephalitis

1

The Arbovirus Encephalitides

H. E. WEBB

Arboviruses are those which in nature can infect blood-sucking arthropods through ingestion of infected vertebrate blood. The virus must be able to invade and multiply in the arthropods' tissue and then be transmitted in their saliva when susceptible vertebrates are bitten. This classification excludes viruses such as myxomatosis and avian pox virus which are only mechanically transmitted by arthropods. At present there are over 300 of these viruses and at least 80 are known to cause human disease. This number increases each year as more studies are undertaken. The arboviruses have been divided into antigenic groups (Casals & Brown 1954; Casals 1957, 1961, 1963) of which A, B, C and California group provide the most recognizable human illness. The Catalogue of Arthropod Borne Viruses of the World (1967) provides an excellent reference book for the distribution of these viruses, the host range of infectivity and the arthropods involved.

The number of clinical cases of encephalitis seen in an arbovirus epidemic will represent only a fraction of the total number of people infected. Clinical involvement extends from the majority who have no detectable illness, through to those who have a short febrile illness, meningitis, encephalitis, and finally a very few who go on to coma and death. It seems likely that less than 1% of the people infected in an epidemic have detectable clinical central nervous system signs but from experimental evidence virus may

3

reach the central nervous system in many patients (Webb et al. 1968b). This could account for the very severe headache suffered in many of these illnesses and also explain some clinical disturbances occurring at a later date such as parkinsonism, epilepsy, dementia and other psychiatric illnesses. For example epilepsia partialis continua and other chronic focal neurological syndromes can be caused by strains of the Russian spring–summer (RSS) encephalitis complex (Asher 1971).

AN ARBOVIRUS ENCEPHALITIS EPIDEMIC

Epidemiologically arbovirus encephalitides are different from other encephalitides discussed in this book because an arbovirus infection will be suspected when cases of encephalitis occur in a group of people who live or work in conditions where they come into contact with a large population of arthropods and a range of vertebrate hosts, both domestic and wild, which could support an arthropod-borne virus. To investigate this situation one needs a clinician, an entomologist and a virologist. The investigation should proceed along the following lines:

The human illness
Attempts must be made to isolate virus from blood, cerebrospinal fluid (CSF) and post-mortem tissues. Acute and convalescent specimens of both serum and CSF must be stored for serological studies. It is important to remember that antibody titres rise later in the CSF than in the blood and a four-fold rise in titre is sometimes detectable in the CSF when it is not detected in blood. The reason for this is that the first serum sample is often taken too late after the onset of the disease to obtain a subsequent four-fold rise in the convalescent serum. A serological survey of antibodies against known neurotropic arboviruses should also be made from the local population who may not have suffered an illness.

4

The arthropods

These should be trapped, identified and processed for virus isolation. If virus is isolated this must be tested against patients' acute and convalescent serum.

The vertebrate hosts

Mammals and birds in the area should be trapped and identified and their ectoparasites should be identified. If arthropods are found they should be processed for virus isolation. The animals should be bled and their sera screened for known arbovirus anti-bodies and against any new virus isolated.

In Table 1 a summary is made of the world-wide distribution of the arboviruses which can cause disturbances of the CNS. As can be seen from the table all these infections except Langat can be acquired naturally. A number have caused laboratory infections but, except in the case of the tick-borne encephalitis (TBE) com-plex, seldom cause encephalitis when acquired in this way. A few have been used in the therapy of malignant disease (T) and have occasionally caused encephalitis when used for this purpose. The arboviruses which cause epidemics of encephalitis are marked 'E'. It is impossible in a table of this nature to cover all the exact areas where these viruses have occurred or the whole range of arthro-pods from which virus has been isolated. The chief vectors of the viruses have been named by species in each case. The main vertebrate hosts in which antibodies are found are also listed and whether they are commonly found naturally (N) or after laboratory infection (L). This does not mean that they are necessarily the effective reservoir for the virus, as the viraemia may never be sufficient to infect biting arthropods. A lot still needs to be done to elucidate which are the real vertebrate virus reservoirs in each disease. One virus of the RSS complex—Central European virus—can also be transmitted to man by goats' milk. In the laboratory there is also evidence of infection from aerosols.

TABLE I

ARBOVIRUSES CAUSING CLINICAL DISTURBANCES IN THE CENTRAL NERVOUS SYSTEM

Virus	Group	Disease in man N	L	T	Geographical distribution	Antibodies found Man	Rodents	Birds	Others	Vector
Bunyamwara	Bunyamwara	+		+*	S. Africa, Uganda, Nigeria	N	L	?	N	Aedes spp.
California	California	E			USA	N	N	N	N	Aedes spp.
Chikungunya	A	+	+		Africa, Thailand, India, Malaya	N	L	—	N	Aedes spp.
Eastern equine	A	E			America, West Indies, Czechoslovakia	N	N	N	N	Culex spp. / Aedes spp.
Ilheus	B	+		+*	Brazil, Trinidad, Colombia, Panama, Honduras, Guatemala	N	N	N	N	Culex spp. / Psorophera spp.
Japanese B	B	E			Japan, Taiwan, Malaya, India, China	N	L	N	N	Culex spp.
Murray Valley	B	E			Australia, New Guinea	N	L	N	N	Culex spp.
Rio Bravo	B	+	+		USA, Mexico	N	—	—	—	?
Tick-borne RSS complex										
Central European	B	E	+		Scandinavia, central Europe	N	N	N	N	Ixodes spp.
Far Eastern	B	E	+	+	USSR	N	N	N	N	Ixodes spp.
Kyasanur Forest	B	+	+		India	N	N	N	N	Haemophylis spp.
Langat	B			+†	Malaya	N	N	N	N	Ixodes spp.
Louping ill	B	+	+		British Isles	N	N	N	N	Ixodes spp.
Negishi	B	+	+		Japan	N	N	N	N	?
West Nile	B	+	+		Egypt, Uganda, Congo (Leo), India, Borneo, USSR, Israel, France	N	N	N	N	Culex spp.
Western equine	A	+	+		USA, S. America	N	N	N	N	Culex spp.
Yellow fever	B	+	+		Africa, S. America	N	L		N	Aedes spp. / Haemagogus spp.

E, epidemic; N, natural; L, laboratory; T, therapeutic.   * Southam and Moore (1951).   † Webb et al. (1966).

CLINICAL SYNDROMES

An arbovirus encephalitis has no particular clinical signs and symptoms which will distinguish it for certain from any other virus encephalitis. The area where the encephalitis occurs and the prevalence of ticks and mosquitoes at that time will determine whether an arbovirus encephalitis is likely.

An arbovirus encephalitis is a biphasic illness in which the first phase, the viraemic phase, may be so mild it is missed (Fig. 1);

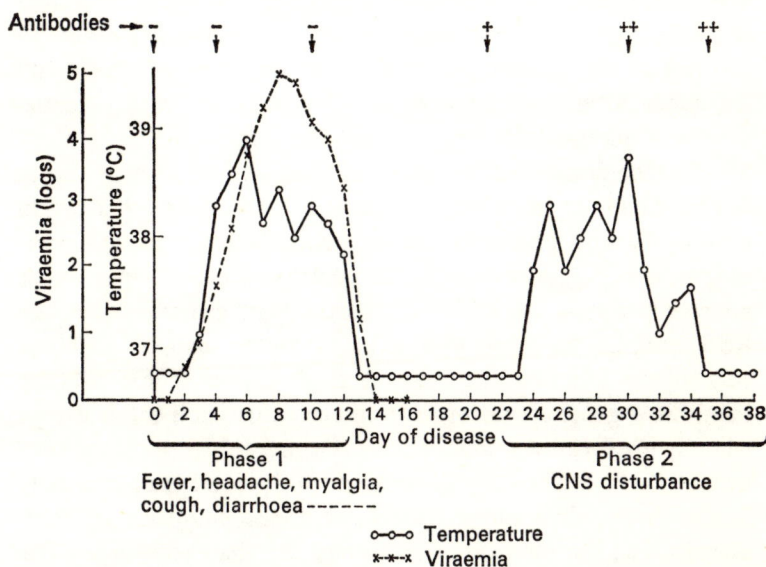

Fig. 1 Clinical and virological findings related to day of disease. Phase 1: fever, headache, myalgia, cough, diarrhoea. Phase 2: CNS disturbance. This Figure has been constructed from studying infections of humans in the field by one of the RSSE virus group: KFD (Webb & Lakshmana Rao 1961). and also of patients being treated in hospital for malignant disease with this virus and the closely related Langat virus (Webb et al. 1966).

however, if a careful history is taken this phase will be apparent. It may be characterized by various combinations of fever, headache, malaise, myalgia, sore throat, skin rashes, tender glands and diarrhoea. At this stage a blood count is likely to show leucopenia and sometimes pancytopenia.

The second phase, which may start only a few days to 3 weeks after the first phase, has 3 types of presentation. The mildest is limited to a second rise in temperature with severe headache, nausea and vomiting. This may go on to the second type, with marked meningism and irritability without localizing signs—meningitis. Lastly, frank encephalitis may develop with or without meningism but with many different neurological signs. These may include convulsions, focal fits, cranial nerve palsies, hemiplegias and paraplegias, ataxia, drowsiness, marked psychosis, retention of urine, coarse tremors, papilloedema, deep coma and death. In the tropics the patient presenting with an acute psychosis and low-grade fever must be assessed very carefully for a potential arbovirus encephalitis. The younger the patient the more likely it is that the disease will be severe and followed by sequelae, if not death. Common sequelae are mental retardation, changes in personality with psychosis and dementia, hemiplegias and paraplegias, epilepsy, post-encephalitic parkinsonism and lower motor neurone paralysis. An infection with the Far Eastern strain of the RSS complex tends to give a lower motor neurone paralysis particularly affecting the cervical cord. Lower motor neurone paralysis is generally uncommon in arbovirus encephalitis except when it involves the cranial nerves. During this phase there may be leucocytosis. The CSF shows pleocytosis and if examined early in the encephalitic phase may show a predominance of polymorphs, but the total count is usually less than 1000/mm³. The CSF sugar is normal or bears a close relationship to the blood sugar. The cells in the CSF become chiefly lymphocytic within the first few days. The CSF protein may be up to 200 mg/100 ml but is usually less than 150 mg/100 ml. A high protein content may persist for a considerable length of time after the illness, in spite of early and apparently complete clinical recovery. The globulin may also be abnormally raised and may persist for a similar period (Webb et al. 1968a). Localized abnormalities may be seen in EEGs and brain scans. The EEGs tend to show a general slow wave activity and epileptiform activity may be seen during the acute illness and also as a sequela. Brain scans showing abnormal focal uptakes have been reported with California (La Crosse) arbovirus infections (Balfour et al. 1973). This may be confused with the type of brain scan abnormalities seen with herpesvirus. It is important to remember that it is usual for all parts of the CNS to show evidence of viral infection on histopathology, although clinical damage associated with such a wide area is not present. The centre of damage is generally around the basal nuclei and brain stem, but the cerebellum, all parts of the cortex, the hippocampus and the spinal cord can show severe changes. The changes are those of any other viral encephalitis with perivascular cuffing, neuronal fall-out, glial nodules and neuronophagia.

TREATMENT

This is basically supportive with particular attention to maintaining the airways and the function of the respiratory and cardiac centres. Full use of intensive care facilities should be made at the earliest signs of respiratory, central or bulbar impairment. Positive pressure ventilation should always be used in preference to negative pressure in order to keep the airways and lungs clear and in case of vomiting during feeding. Surprising recoveries with a reasonable standard of life can occur even after months of unconsciousness. As those who die have intense oedema of the brain and cord, sometimes associated with marked papilloedema during life, it is completely justifiable to use steroids as antioedematous agents to reduce intracranial pressure. If used for this purpose they should be given in large doses but only for a short time. The object is to reduce oedema and the fall-out of further neurones from anoxia due to ischaemia. Antiviral agents have not been tried in a sufficient number of cases to assess their value. To date there have been no spectacular successes. Anticonvulsive drugs may be needed in the post-encephalitic phase, as may drugs to treat psychotic and schizophrenic-like states. The most common postencephalitic psychological problem is acute depression, for which both electroconvulsive therapy and ordinary antidepressants,

9

tricyclics and monoamine oxidase inhibitors, may be very useful. This aspect of the convalescent period is frequently forgotten not only in cases of arbovirus encephalitis but in other encephalitides and other conditions which damage CNS tissue. First-class nursing is absolutely essential to prevent bed sores and flexor or other contractions developing, as is intensive physiotherapy and a good diet to build up the muscle loss suffered during the disease.

It is this type of encephalitis which good public health measures and education of the population ought to be able to prevent. A major object of any medical treatise on human disease is to try and put forward a method of preventing the occurrence of the illness, particularly in the case of virus encephalitis where the treatment remains almost entirely a supportive matter rather than a direct attack on the virus itself. It is therefore of particular importance in the arbovirus encephalitides to examine carefully the factors which are involved in human infections.

FACTORS INVOLVED IN HUMAN INFECTIONS WITH ARBOVIRUSES

This problem has been examined in considerable detail by Smith (1962, 1964a, b). In the arthropod-borne zoonoses the virus is maintained in an arthropod between one vertebrate and the next, man being involved incidentally.

Host viraemia
For successful arthropod infection, the degree of the viraemia in the host must equal or exceed that required for infection of the arthropod species concerned.

Vertebrate population factors
From the two preceding points it can be seen that for an infection to be established and continued there must not only be a supply of susceptible hosts, frequently rodents and birds, but also a continuous replenishment of a population which is non-immune. It is quite clear that the number of successful transmissions of

virus is proportional to the host population which is non-immune. A high incidence of circulating antibody prevents viraemia and therefore rules out reinfection of biting arthropods. In some parts of the world, such as Singapore and Malaya where Japanese B encephalitis is present all the year round, there is an adequate renewal of the non-immune vertebrate population for reinfection to take place. In other parts of the world this clearly is not the case, epidemics occurring only when the level of susceptible hosts is increased.

The climate and microclimate
The type of climate and microclimate which is present affects the breeding and feeding activity of both mosquitoes and ticks. Low temperatures reduce the biting and breeding activity of mosquitoes (Walker et al. 1942), whereas high humidity increases a mosquito's life span. Virus multiplication in the mosquito is to a certain extent temperature-dependent. The temperature of arthropod tissue is only slightly above that of the environment. At low temperatures virus may persist in a mosquito but not multiply sufficiently to cause reinfection. Arthropod transmission can only take place if there has been adequate multiplication of virus within the arthropod to cause reinfection when it bites. However, short periods of high temperature can drastically shorten the incubation period (Bates & Roca-Garcia 1946). The tick-borne viruses are not so important in this respect, as intervals between feeding are likely to be longer than the incubation period. As regards feeding habits in ticks, Smorodintsev (1958) showed that *Ixodes persulcatus*, the vector of Far Eastern encephalitis, starts biting at a temperature of about 3–4°C, reaches a maximum at 10–12°C and decreases in activity above 18°C. The humidity requirement of different species of ticks determines their distribution. For example, *Ixodes ricinus*, transmitter of encephalitis, requires a very high humidity for its development. In the British Isles this type of environment is found in thick grasses and rushes on poorly drained land, whereas in Europe it occurs on the floor of deciduous and mixed forests. Ticks can pass on a virus infection transovarially, so that the next generation can become infected to

such an extent that they are able to cause infection in further vertebrate hosts.

Human behaviour

Man, at the present time, can alter his environment very quickly. By air he can travel within a few hours from areas of scrubland to areas of bush and thick vegetation. He therefore exposes himself in each situation to the possibility of different infections from a wide range of biting arthropods and the arboviruses they may carry. Those who travel quickly from one type of area to another in this way, e.g. to give advice on various projects such as agricultural or hydroelectric problems, run the risk of picking up arbovirus infections to which the local populations of the areas they visit have a very high level of antibody. Man will also change the ecology of areas quickly, e.g. he can clear forests or make fertile pastures out of deserts. In doing this he changes very significantly the type of vertebrate likely to live there and the type of arthropod likely to be present. If the local population remains and these other natural factors change, these people will become susceptible to epidemics of new arbovirus infections induced by the man-made change. Man can, therefore, control his environment, should it become necessary, by removing areas suitable for breeding mosquitoes or killing vertebrates thought to be reservoirs of virus disease. Frequently this is not possible and it therefore remains true that the best way to avoid getting an arbovirus infection is to avoid getting bitten.

DIRECTION OF MODERN RESEARCH

At the time of writing a new epidemic of Murray Valley encephalitis is occurring in the Murray Valley itself. Experts are trying to find out the reason for this. One major interest lies in the role that birds, migrating to and through this area, may have had in starting this epidemic. Research is also going on into the effect of the recent increase in rainfall which has improved the conditions for mosquito breeding. It is of paramount importance to try and find out the reasons for this new virus outbreak. It raises the fascinating question of where viruses of the arbovirus encephalitides survive in the non-epidemic seasons. Reeves (1961) discussed in detail the possibilities to account for the 'overwintering' of viruses. Long-term survival of western equine, St Louis and Japanese B encephalitis viruses has been found in birds (Webster & Clow 1936; Slavin 1943; Reeves et al. 1958) and Japanese B and Venezuelan equine encephalitis virus in hibernating bats (Corristan et al. 1956; Lamotte 1958). Western equine virus can overwinter in garter snakes to an extent that the viraemia in these reptiles the following spring was great enough to infect mosquitoes fed on them. Recently Watts et al. (1973) have proved that transovarial transmission of the La Crosse virus (California encephalitis group) occurs in the mosquito *Aedes triseriatus* and have suggested that this is the overwintering mechanism for this arbovirus in the northern United States. Burgdorfer and Varma (1967) have reviewed the fascinating work on the transovarial passage of virus in tick replication. Transovarial passage of virus is unequivocally confirmed with the viruses of the tick-borne encephalitis complex. These viruses can also survive under natural conditions of hibernation for over 100 days in engorged larvae of *Ixodes ricinus* (Rehacek 1960). Virus can survive in the brains of humans for months (Freyman 1957) and in rodents for months and years (Price 1966; Goverdham & Anderson 1972). It is with this in mind that one must consider the long-term pathological effects of arboviruses on the CNS as demonstrated in epilepsia partialis continua. The arboviruses have a definite capacity to produce excessive glial proliferation (Zlotnik 1968; Illavia & Webb 1969, 1970, 1972; Precious et al. 1974). It seems possible that this may be a primary proliferative effect on the glial cells by the virus. Tanaka and Southam (1962) have shown that encephalitogenic arboviruses can enhance tumour formation in experimental animals. In the acute encephalitic illness itself, it is not yet clear how much damage is due to the primary cytolytic effect of the virus in the CNS and how much is due to the allergic response of the host itself. This problem of the allergic response in virus disease is reviewed by Webb and Hall (1972). Virus isolation from cases of arbovirus encephalitis is unusual unless the patient dies. This is because the illness starts after the viraemic phase has finished and antibodies are present in the blood. Experiments in monkeys using Kyasanur Forest disease virus (TBE complex) have shown that during this second phase there is virus present in muscle as well as CNS tissue (Webb 1961). Similar studies have been done during the paralytic phase in mice infected with Langat (TBE complex) and West Nile viruses. In both incidences virus has been recovered from muscle tissue (Bateman 1974). It might be justifiable, therefore, to take muscle biopsies from human beings during the early paralytic phase of a viral illness to try and isolate the causative agent. If this is done, both co-cultivation techniques of muscle with a suitable cell culture line as well as direct inoculation into suckling mice should be used to achieve virus isolation.

A great deal of work is in progress on the structure of these viruses and as a result they are being reclassified. The name 'arbovirus' should be used for viruses having a biological cycle in both arthropods and vertebrates but it should be stressed that this terminology has only an ecological significance. A structural classification has been proposed by the 1970 vertebrate virus sub-committee on the nomenclature of viruses, giving the name togaviruses (from the latin *toga*, a cloak) to arboviruses having taxonomic characters like those of the serological groups A and B (Andrewes 1970). Enough information has been compiled recently on the characteristic structures of these viruses to rename Group A as alphaviruses and Group B as flavoviruses, the latter name being related to their connection with yellow (*flavus*) fever. It would appear that the arthropod-borne members of the togavirus family are relatively small spherical RNA viruses with a size range of 38–89 nm for the alphaviruses and 30–55 nm for the flavoviruses. This is much smaller for example than the Bunyamwara super-group which range in size from 60 to 130 nm (Holmes 1971). This group is likely to be renamed bunyavirus (Porterfield et al. 1975).

The toga virion has a spherical core which is wrapped in an envelope containing projections on its surfaces. There does not seem to be a correlation with this structure and arthropod transmission. There are many non-arbovirus members of the toga group, e.g. rubella, lactic dehydrogenase virus and others. The whole subject is excellently reviewed by Horzinek (1973) who goes into great detail on the differences in external and internal structures of these viruses. As yet no obvious relationship of structure to potential encephalitogenesis has been forthcoming but it is through this type of work that some common denominator may appear in the structure of viruses which is related to their particular capacity to produce CNS damage.

Interesting work has been published recently showing electron microscopic pictures of the way arboviruses may get into the brain from the capillaries using Semliki Forest virus as a model. The blood–brain barrier is normally impermeable to particles of arbovirus size, but it is suggested that by a process of capillary endothelial cell pinocytosis (phagocytosis) the virus is taken in and delivered to the basement membrane from where the virus is spread by a pressure gradient into the extracellular spaces. The cell membranes of certain cells, especially neurones, appear to react to the presence of virus by forming further phagocytotic vesicles and thus absorbing the virus into the cell. After multiplication the virus particles are delivered again to the cell membrane in vesicles and released into the extracellular spaces and so the process continues. The other suggestion made is that the virus travels in and out of the brain phagocytosed in blood cells (Pathak & Webb 1974).

So it can be seen that there are many aspects of arbovirus infections which are fascinating to study. Many are relatively easy and safe to work with and much interesting work will be accomplished in this field over the next few years.

REFERENCES

Andrews, C. H. (1970) Generic names of viruses of vertebrates. *Virology*, **40**, 1070.

Asher, D. (1971) Focal neurological disease with chronic encephalitis in children and in an experimental primate model. *13th int. Congr. Pediatrics, Vienna*, III, 379.

Balfour, H. H., Siem, R. A., Bauer, H. & Quie, P. G. (1973) California arbovirus (La Crosse) infections. I. Clinical and laboratory findings in 66 children with meningoencephalitis. *Pediatrics, Springfield*, **52**, 680.

Bateman, S. E. (1974) Personal communication.

Bates, M. & Roca-Garcia, M. (1946) The development of the virus of yellow fever in haemogogus mosquitoes. *Am. J. trop. Med.*, **26**, 585.

Burgdofer, W. & Varma, M. G. R. (1967) Trans-stadial and transovarial development of disease agents in arthropods. *Ann. Rev. Entomol.*, **12**, 347.

Casals, J. (1957) The arthropod-borne group of animal viruses. *Trans. N.Y. Acad. Sci., Series 2*, **19**, 219.

Casals, J. (1963) New developments in the classification of arthropod-borne animal viruses. *Proc. VII int. Congr. trop. Med. Malaria*, Part A, 13.

Casals, J. (1961) Procedures for identification of arthropod-borne viruses. *Bull. Wld Hlth Org.*, **24**, 723.

Casals, J. & Brown, L. V. (1954) Haemagglutination with arthropod-borne viruses. *J. exp. Med.*, **99**, 429.

Corristan, E. C., Lamotte, L. C. & Smith, D. G. (1956) Susceptibility of rats to certain encephalitis viruses. *Fedn Proc. Fedn Am. Socs exp. Biol.*, **15**, 1.

Freymann, R. (1957) The virus encephalitides in the Soviet Union and in central Europe. I. Spring–summer tick encephalitis. *Ber. Osteur. Inst. Berl.*, **28**, 34.

Goverdham, M. L. & Anderson, C. R. (1972) The reaction of *Mus platythrix* to Kyasanur Forest disease virus. *Indian J. med. Res.*, **60**, 1002.

Holmes, I. H. (1971) Morphological similarity of Bunyamwera super-group viruses. *Virology*, **43**, 708.

Horzinek, M. C. (1973) Comparative aspects of togaviruses. *J. gen. Virol.*, **20**, 87.

Illavia, S. J. & Webb, H. E. (1969) Maintenance of encephalitogenic viruses by non-neuronal cerebral cells. *Br. med. J.*, **i**, 94.

Illavia, S. J. & Webb, H. E. (1970) An encephalitogenic virus (Langat) in mice. Isolation and persistence in cultures of brains after intraperitoneal infection with the virus. *Lancet*, **ii**, 284.

Illavia, S. J. & Webb, H. E. (1972) The effect of encephalitogenic viruses on tissue culture of non-neuronal cells of mouse and human brain. *Neurology, Minneap.*, **22**, 619.

Lamotte, L. C. (1958) Japanese B encephalitis in bats during simulated hibernation. *Am. J. Hyg.*, **67**, 101.

Pathak, S. & Webb, H. E. (1974) Possible mechanisms for the transport of Semliki Forest virus into and within mouse brain. An electron microscopical study. *J. neurol. Sci.*, **23**, 175.

Porterfield, J. S., Casals, J., Chumakov, M. P., Gaidamovich, S. Ya., Hannoun, C., Holmes, I. H., Horninek, M. C., Mussgay, M. & Russell, P. K. (1975) Bunyaviruses and Bunyviridae. *Intervirology*, in the press.

Precious, S. W., Webb, H. E. & Bowen, E. T. W. (1974) Isolation and persistence of Chikungunya virus in cultures of mouse brain cells. *J. gen. Virol.*, **23**, 271.

Price, W. H. (1966) Chronic disease and virus persistence in mice inoculated with KFD virus. *Virology*, **29**, 679.

Reeves, W. C. (1961) Overwintering of arthropod-borne viruses. *Prog. med. Virol.*, **3**, 59.

Reeves, W. C., Hutson, G. A., Bellamy, R. E. & Scrivani, R. P. (1958) Chronic latent infections of birds with western equine encephalomyelitis virus. *Proc. Soc. exp. Biol., N.Y.*, **97**, 733.

Rehacek, J. (1960) Experimental hibernation of the tick-borne encephalitis virus in engorged larvae of the tick *Ixodes ricinus* L. *Acta virol.*, **4**, 106.

Slavin, H. B. (1943) Persistence of the virus of St Louis encephalitis in the central nervous system of mice for over 5 months. *J. Bact.*, **46**, 113.

Smith, C. E. G. (1962) Ticks and viruses. *Symp. Zool. Soc. Lond.*, **6**, 199.

Smith, C. E. G. (1964a) Factors in the transmission of virus infections from animals to man. *Lect. scient. Basis Med.*, **8**, 125.

Smith, C. E. G. (1964b) Factors influencing the behaviour of viruses in their arthropodian hosts. *2nd Symp. Br. Soc. Parasitol.*, 31.

Smorodintsev, A. A. (1958) Tick-borne spring–summer encephalitis. *Prog. med. Virol.*, **1**, 400.

Southam, C. M. & Moore, A. E. (1951) West Nile, Ilheus and Bunyamwera virus infections in man. *Am. J. trop. Med.*, **31**, 724.

Tanaka, S. & Southam, C. M. (1962) Joint action of West Nile virus and chemical carcinogens in production of papillomas in mice. *J. natn Cancer Inst.*, **29**, 721.

Walker, A. S., Meyers, E., Woodhill, A. R. & McCullough, R. N. (1942) Dengue fever. *Med. J. Aust.*, **2**, 223.

Watts, D. M., Pantuwatana, S., De Foliart, G. R., Yull, T. M. & Thompson, W. H. (1973) Transovarial transmission of La Crosse virus (California encephalitis group) in the mosquito, *Aedes triseriatus*. *Science, N.Y.*, **82**, 1140.

Webb, H. E. (1961) Kyasanur Forest disease in animals and man. D. M. Thesis, Oxford University.

Webb, H. E., Connolly, J. H., Kane, F. F., O'Reilly, K. J. & Simpson, D. I. H. (1968a) Laboratory infections with louping-ill with associated encephalitis. *Lancet*, **ii**, 255.

Webb, H. E. & Hall, J. G. (1972) An assessment of the role of the allergic response in the pathogenesis of viral diseases. *Symp. Soc. gen. Microbiol.*, **22**, 383.

Webb, H. E. & Lakshmana Rao, R. (1961) Kyasanur Forest disease. *Trans. R. Soc. trop. Med. Hyg.*, **55**, 284.

Webb, H. E., Wetherley-Mein, G., Smith, C. E. G. & McMahon, D. (1966) Leukaemia and neoplastic processes treated with Langat and Kyasanur Forest disease viruses: A clinical and laboratory study of 28 patients. *Br. med. J.*, **i**, 258.

Webb, H. E., Wight, D. G. D., Platt, G. S. & Smith, C. E. G. (1968b) Langat virus encephalitis in mice. 1. The effect of the administration of specific antiserum. *J. Hyg., Camb.*, **60**, 343.

Webster, L. T. & Clow, A. D. (1936) Experimental encephalitis (St Louis type) in mice with high inborn resistance. *J. exp. Med.*, **63**, 827.

Zlotnik, I. (1968) Reaction of astrocytes to acute virus infections of the central nervous system. *Br. J. exp. Path.*, **49**, 555.

2

The General Nature of Viral Encephalitis in the United Kingdom

MAURICE LONGSON

According to the *Sydenham Society Lexicon* of 1883, the term encephalitis is used to describe inflammation of the substance of the brain, as distinct from its membranes. The *Lexicon* goes on to emphasize that encephalitis can assail the brain tissue generally, or it can be confined to one spot of the organ. There is no reason why we should today have to change this good, if simple, definition of the disease.

Encephalitis, or brain fever, has been a common 'foot of the bed' diagnosis for many centuries; there are on record accounts of many epidemics, such as Sydenham's febris comatosa of 1673 and the outbreaks of nona in Italy at the end of the last century. It is of interest to note that for many years, encephalitis was believed to be particularly related to influenza. Notwithstanding this often-quoted association, the cause of encephalitis for long remained a total mystery, except perhaps in the case of rabies, where experimental proof of communicability became available in the first decade of the nineteenth century (Zinke, quoted by Johnson 1965).

Rabies certainly represents a landmark in the history of infectious diseases of the brain and Louis Pasteur should perhaps be honoured as the founder of neurovirology, although it will be remembered that Pasteur himself only surmised about the viral nature of the rabies agent. Nevertheless, it was again with rabies that viruses first made their entry into the conscious world of neurologists when, in 1903, Remlinger demonstrated that the disease was caused by a filterable microbial agent.

Another epoch in the birth of neurovirology was undoubtedly seen in the early 1920s. This was to be an era of important discoveries. During the 5 preceding years, Von Economo's epidemic encephalitis had spread its rather fearsome grip across Europe, North America and Japan. The evidence strongly suggested a communicable nature and there is no doubt that the disease bore many of the hallmarks of a virus infection. Many different microbial agents became incriminated, but the reports which were to have the greatest impact were those by Levaditi and Harvier (1920) and Doerr and Schnabel (1922). It was stated that a virus, later proved to be *Herpesvirus simplex*, could be isolated from cerebrospinal fluids or from necropsy brains. Today we do not really know whether these twenty or so isolates were accidental contaminants and represent what some have called 'a virological misadventure', or whether indeed encephalitis lethargica was a variant of herpes encephalitis.

The gradual and almost total loss of interest in neurovirology which followed the decline of encephalitis lethargica in the mid-1920s was only re-awakened, 10 years later, by a remarkable outbreak of encephalitis which occurred in Illinois. Already, in 1925, Takagi (1925) had isolated an insect-borne virus from patients with Japanese B encephalitis, but the reports had passed largely unnoticed in the Occident. In 1933, Muckenfuss et al. in St Louis, Illinois, proved that the American outbreak was also caused by a similar agent. A further epidemic occurred in the USA in 1937 and altogether there were well over 2000 cases, with a case mortality rate of about 20%.

When war broke out in Europe in 1939, the details of the recent American experience were making an impact in London. There was still a vivid memory of the Von Economo epidemic which had waxed in Europe during the First World War and it was not surprising that the War Cabinet ordered a surveillance of encepha-

litis in England and Wales. The cause of encephalitis lethargica
had remained obscure and there was the not unreasonable fear
that war conditions might favour the introduction of insect-borne
encephalitis into the United Kingdom. The surveillance was
undertaken by two people—Professor James McIntosh, who took
responsibility for animal inoculations, and the distinguished
neuropathologist, Dr J. G. Greenfield, who examined the histological preparations from necropsy material submitted to him
from all over the country.

Greenfield thus accumulated a vast experience and his observations commanded widespread respect. Indeed, we owe much to
Greenfield and, with only minor modifications made in the light
of current knowledge, his classification of encephalitis remains
valid to this day (Greenfield 1950).

Using the language of the *Sydenham Lexicon* and confining our
attention to diseases 'of the substance of the brain', we can classify
viral encephalitis as (*a*) acute polioclastic encephalitis (acute viral
panencephalitis), (*b*) diffuse perivascular leucoencephalitis and (*c*)
chronic viral neuropathies ('slow' virus encephalopathies).

ACUTE POLIOCLASTIC ENCEPHALITIS

These are acute proven, or assumed, viral infections which predominantly affect the grey matter (Gk: πολιός =grey). In many
cases the white matter may also be involved, thus producing a
panencephalitis. Neuronal damage is an invariable finding, there
is an acute inflammatory response and it is believed that brain
damage is in the main the direct result of viral replication within
the affected tissue itself. Demyelination is not a feature. Acute
virus encephalitis can be either epidemic or sporadic.

Epidemic viral encephalitis includes those diseases caused by
various members of the genuses Alphavirus (arbovirus group A)
and flavoviruses (arbovirus group B) and those caused by the different human Enteroviruses: polio, coxsackie and echo. The most
common cause of sporadic viral encephalitis is probably *Herpes-*

virus simplex (Editorial, *British Medical Journal* 1973) but other recognized aetiological agents include *Herpesvirus varicellae* (Juel-Jensen & MacCallum 1972), cytomegalovirus (Dorfman 1973), *Herpesvirus simiae* (B virus) (Hartley 1966), lymphocytic chorio-meningitis virus (Ackermann 1973), mumps virus, *Adenovirus hominis* (Roos et al. 1972), encephalomyocarditis virus (Gajdusek 1955), rabies virus and louping ill virus (Illis & Gostling 1972). For the sake of completeness, mention can be made of Rickettsiacae which, although not true viruses, are considered to be infrequent causes of 'viral' encephalitis. These include *Chlamydia psittaci* and *C. trachomatis* group G (lymphogranuloma venereum agent), *Rickettsia rickettsi* and *R. prowazeki*, and the agent of cat-scratch disease.

Agents such as Epstein-Barr virus, measles virus, *Orthomyxovirus influenza* and rubella virus are known to be involved in the aetiology of post-infectious encephalomyelitis (see below) but there is now some evidence that they may also cause true acute viral encephalitis, with actual and active presence of the virus in the central nervous system (CNS) itself (Flewett & Hoult 1958; Termeulen et al. 1972; Lascelles et al. 1973).

DIFFUSE PERIVASCULAR LEUCOENCEPHALITIS

Often described as an acute post-infectious encephalomyelitis, this form of encephalopathy is characterized by a predominantly white matter disease revealing conduction defects caused by localized or widespread demyelination. Acute haemorrhagic encephalitis is probably an extreme form of the condition. It is said that the pathogenesis is 'allergic', following autoimmune sensitization to brain antigens or to encephalitogenic factors. Present knowledge does not suggest that actual virus invasion of nervous tissue is necessary for the initiation of the disease process. Symptoms referable to the nervous system usually appear 10 to 14 days (extremes 2 to 25 days) after infection of other organs by agents such as vaccinia virus, measles virus, rubella virus, *Herpesvirus varicellae*, cytomegalovirus, Epstein-Barr virus (infectious mononucleosis), *Orthomyxovirus influenza* and, indeed, many other respiratory viruses.

The distinction between acute virus encephalitis and acute post-infectious encephalomyelitis may be extremely difficult unless the causative agent can be identified in biopsy tissue or cerebrospinal fluid. Later, during convalescence, measurement of specific antibody in the cerebrospinal fluid and a calculation of the serum: CSF antibody ratio may help. It is the author's experience that there is never any change in the ratio of specific antibody unless the suspected virus has been directly involved in the actual nervous tissue disease process. In diffuse perivascular encephalitis, there may be a rise of specific antibody in the serum, but this will not be reflected by any significant change in the CSF antibody level.

CHRONIC VIRAL ENCEPHALOPATHIES

Greenfield (1950) actually described 4 types of encephalitis, but he clearly foresaw the possibility that his so-called 'inclusion body encephalitis' and Van Bogaert's subacute sclerosing pan- or leuco-encephalitis (SSPE) were one and the same condition.

The chronic viral or 'slow virus' encephalitis, as usually grouped, presents as a heterogenous collection of diseases. There is little doubt that a lot more light will be shed on this classification during the next few years. It is perhaps useful at this stage to subdivide the group into 3 sub-groups and limit ourselves to known diseases of man:

1. *Encephalopathies involving an inflammatory reaction in the brain*
   Subacute sclerosing panencephalitis (SSPE)
   Progressive multifocal leucoencephalopathy (PML)
2. *Congenital encephalopathies following in utero infection of the fetus*
   Rubella and cytomegalovirus encephalopathies

3. *Subacute spongiform encephalopathies with no inflammatory reaction*
Kuru
Jakob–Creutzfeldt disease
Alzheimer's pre-senile dementia (possibly)

The nosology and the aetiology of the diseases which will be presented in detail during the course of this book have been discussed briefly and we can now consider the magnitude of the various problems as we see them in the United Kingdom. This presentation of the epidemiological figures will be limited to the incidence of the various forms of acute viral encephalitis seen in this country during the past 7 to 8 years. Analysis of the figures over the past 25 years gives no reason to suppose that the epidemiological picture has changed since the Greenfield study already described.

There is little doubt that there is gross under-reporting of cases of encephalitis. It is the author's experience that most cases of viral encephalitis are never notified to any official, or unofficial, authority and there are reasons to believe that this is a national problem. What is more, one has the nasty feeling that in many, if not most, of the notified cases the diagnosis of 'encephalitis' will not withstand critical examination. The diagnostic criteria used are often much too lax and many cases of headache or vague disturbance of cerebration, with or without pyrexia and other systemic symptoms, are erroneously reported. The figures to be presented should therefore be treated with the circumspection they deserve.

The sources of information about the epidemiology of viral encephalitis in the United Kingdom are three-fold:

1. *The Registrar General's Statistical Reviews*, which provide figures for England and Wales. The tables are compiled from certified causes of death as entered on Medical Death Certificates, or from Notifications of Infectious Diseases under the Health Services and Public Health Act 1968. It is noteworthy that 'encephalitis' is one of the 'notifiable diseases' and as such, all new cases should by law be reported to the health authority. As

it has been said, the law is not observed and enforcement is impossible.

2. *The Communicable Diseases Report* (*CDR*) published by the Epidemiological Research Laboratory of the Public Health Laboratory Service Board. This document collects information voluntarily submitted by diagnostic laboratories throughout England and Wales. It also includes cases from Scotland reported by the Department of Infectious Diseases, Glasgow. Many contributing laboratories report assiduously, others indifferently. The Report provides very accurate information about positive isolation of infective agents but the accuracy of the clinical diagnosis it reports is limited by the quality of the information given by the clinician in his original request to the laboratory.

The CDR cannot, of course, provide any information about the very many cases of genuine encephalitis where laboratory tests either have not been undertaken or have not revealed the nature of the causative agent.

3. *Private registers*, managed by workers with particular research interests in certain areas of neurovirology, such as the SSPE Register (Dick 1973), the Herpes Encephalitis Register organized by the Herpes Encephalitis Working Party (Liversedge et al. 1972) and the Jakob–Creutzfeldt Disease Register kept by Professor Matthews (see p. 146).

Table 2 gives figures obtained from the Registrar General's

TABLE 2

DEATHS AND NOTIFICATIONS OF ENCEPHALITIS
IN THE UNITED KINGDOM 1967–71

Disease	Deaths	Notifications
Viral encephalitis	385*	—
Encephalitis and encephalomyelitis	482*	—
Encephalitis (infectious)	—	563†
Encephalitis (post-infectious)	—	471†

* Certified cause of death in Registrar General's Statistical Tables.
† Notifications of disease in Registrar General's Statistical Tables.

Tables for the five-year period ending December 1971 and includes both Certified Causes of Death and notification of infectious diseases. In the International Classification of Diseases, the terms 'viral encephalitis' (ICD Nos. 062-063-064-065) and 'encephalitis and encephalomyelitis' (ICD No. 323) are widely separated into different classes, but according to the Rules of Classification, (World Health Organisation 1967), there should not be any double entries. It thus appears as though there are about 175 encephalitis deaths per year in England and Wales. There is no way of correlating the 'death' and 'notification' figures, but there are, as might be expected, slightly more notified cases (about 200) than deaths each year.

Table 3 attempts to list the viruses which might have caused the

TABLE 3

CAUSES OF ACUTE ENCEPHALITIS

Cause	Deaths*	Notifications†	Communicable diseases report
Adenovirus	—		16
Arbovirus	2		0
Enterovirus	26		200
Herpes simplex	105‡	49	242
Infectious mono-nucleosis	—	5	§
Lymphocytic chorio-meningitis	—		6
Measles	—	41	82
Mumps	—	7	234
Poliomyelitis	4	66	‖
Rabies	2		0
Rubella	—	3¶	0
Varicella	—	24	10

* Certified cause of death in Registrar General's Statistical Tables.

† Notification of Disease in Registrar General's Statistical Tables.

‡ Includes all deaths attributable to herpes simplex virus.

§ Causative agent cannot be isolated.

‖ Very many virus isolates, but majority vaccine strains and probably of very little significance.

¶ One year only; no figures prior to 1971.

cases of encephalitis during the same 5-year period. In the column headed 'Deaths', the figures entered represent cases where, in the Registrar General's Tables, the cause of the fatal encephalitis is directly attributable to one of a few specifically mentioned viruses. Under the heading 'Notifications' are listed the numbers of cases of poliomyelitis and the number of cases of encephalitis which were notified and described as being complications of certain specified infectious diseases. The figures do not distinguish between cases of acute viral encephalitis and post-infectious encephalomyelitis. In the column headed 'CDR' are entered the number of times certain viruses were incriminated by a laboratory as the cause of diseases in circumstances where a *clinical* diagnosis of encephalitis appeared possible. For the purpose of this review, study is limited to cases where the laboratory evidence resides, at least in part, in virus isolation; serological results have not been considered. The figures require careful interpretation. As has already been underlined, the quality of the *clinical* diagnosis in the CDR figures is open to some criticism and, furthermore, the reported virus might not necessarily have been isolated from brain or CSF. It is by no means certain that an aetiological role in CNS disease can be ascribed to a virus isolated from a non-CNS specimen. For example, the isolation of *Herpesvirus simplex* from a throat or mouth swab cannot, by itself, confirm the diagnosis of herpes encephalitis, however convincing may be the evidence of cerebral involvement. Similarly, in a patient with headaches, meningism and faecal excretion of enterovirus, the diagnosis of enterovirus encephalitis must remain in doubt until more positive evidence of actual CNS infection becomes available. Similar care is required in the interpretation of serological results, unless these are obtained from the examination of the CSF.

Space does not permit a critical examination of all the CDR figures but a few examples will illustrate the difficulties. In the 5-year period 1967–71, there were well over 200 isolations of enteroviruses from cases of 'encephalitis'. It would appear that very few of the isolates came from CNS specimens. For example, in 1971 and 1972, the predominant enteroviruses were coxsackie-virus B5 and B4 respectively. In 1971, there were 13 isolates of coxsackievirus B5 from cases of encephalitis, none of which were obtained from nervous tissue or fluid. Of the 12 coxsackievirus B4 in cases of encephalitis during 1972, only 1 appears to have been obtained from CNS material. Similarly, in the same 5-year period, there were 16 cases of encephalitis ascribed to adenoviruses, but only in 2 of these cases were the isolates obtained from CSF. (Amongst 39 cases of possible adenovirus meningitis, only 2 isolates came from CSF.) The viruses involved were either adenovirus type 1 or adenovirus type 6. Symptomless excretion of coxsackieviruses and respiratory infection with adenoviruses are almost facts of life—the mere presence of these agents in a throat swab or faeces does not give them an aetiological role in CNS disease.

Measles, mumps and varicella present similar problems. Between 1967 and 1971, there were 1232 isolates of measles virus from patients with measles. Of these patients, 82 presented with symptoms suggesting an encephalitis. During the same 5-year period, there were in all 1866 isolates of mumps virus, of which 234 cases presented with encephalitis, 898 with meningitis and 115 with 'other CNS symptoms'. If we look at the 1971 figures in more detail, we find that 114 alleged cases of mumps meningo-encephalitis with positive virus isolation were reported, but that in only 29 of these was the virus isolated from the CSF. There were 506 isolates of *Herpesvirus varicella* during 1967–71 and in 10 of these cases, a clinical diagnosis of encephalitis was reported. Meningitis and 'other CNS symptoms' were reported in 23 and 28 cases, respectively. During 1971, there were 17 reported cases of varicella meningoencephalitis, but the virus was isolated from CSF in only a single instance.

Finally, I will turn my attention to herpes encephalitis, which has been said to be the most common form of sporadic encephalitis occurring in temperate climates.

According to the Registrar General's figures, there were 105 deaths attributable to *Herpesvirus simplex* (ICD No. 054) in the years 1967–71 (Table 3). The figure does not, of course, state the nature of the organ primarily affected by the virus, but with the exception of neonatal herpes, itself a rare condition in the United

Kingdom, herpes encephalitis is certainly the commonest form of fatal herpetic infection and the figure of 105 could be an indication of the incidence of fatal herpes encephalitis. On the other hand, in the same period, only 49 cases of encephalitis secondary to herpes simplex virus infection were notified to the Medical Officers of Health (Table 3). Because of the very nature of herpes febrilis and of the general inadequacy of the notifications of encephalitis, this figure of 49 is probably irrelevant in any evaluation of the frequency of the disease.

The CDR reports are possibly of more interest. In the 5-year period, 242 cases of herpes encephalitis were recorded. On behalf of the Working Party on Herpes Encephalitis, Dr F. O. Mac-Callum and the author have communicated with the laboratories and clinicians who were primarily responsible for these 242 cases. Using strict criteria for the diagnosis (recognition of virus in CNS material, or a strong histopathological evidence of acute necrotising encephalitis, supported by serological evidence of infection), it was felt that the diagnosis could only be upheld in about 20% of cases (57 out of 242). At the same time, the Working Party was compiling its own register of cases. Direct contact with the membership of the British Association of Neurologists, the Society of British Neurological Surgeons, the British Neuropathological Society, the Society for the Study of Infectious Diseases and with virologists in the various centres of the British Isles has been a very fruitful exercise. In the 7-year period 1966–72, 99 cases of herpes encephalitis, diagnosed according to the same strict criteria, have been entered on the register. There is an equal distribution in the sexes and the disease appears to occur in all age groups.

There is no doubt that the Working Party figures provide a significant underestimate of the frequency of herpes encephalitis. The diagnosis is substantiated in only the fairly major centres and many cases of the disease must go unrecognized, undiagnosed and unnotified. As a working hypothesis, it can, however, be suggested that up to 50 cases of herpes encephalitis occur in the United Kingdom each year and that about half of these could be recognized in sufficient time for possibly effective chemotherapy.

In conclusion, it will have become abundantly clear that we have, to say the least, only a rudimentary and fragmentary knowledge of the epidemiology of viral encephalitis in the United Kingdom. As Dr Illis and others will be emphasizing elsewhere in this book, we now have at our disposal a number of ways of interfering with the natural progress of these extremely severe diseases, but a sound appraisal of the impact of these methods will require a precise knowledge of the epidemiology of encephalitis. It is therefore most important that we should improve our methods of surveillance. This is not an easy task, and as an immediate measure, one would like to encourage the conscientious yielding of information to the various specialist registers which are already in existence, or which may in future make their appearance.

I am deeply grateful to Mrs Enid Vernon, of the Epidemiological Research Laboratory, Central Public Health Laboratory, London, for the abundant provision of figures used in this review and to Dr T. Pollock, Director of the Epidemiological Research Laboratory, for permission to use data compiled by his Department, and for having read the manuscript.

REFERENCES

Ackermann, R. (1973) In *Lymphocytic Choriomeningitis Virus*, ed. Lehmann-Grube, F. Berlin: Springer Verlag.

Communicable Disease Report (Four-weekly virus report) London: Public Health Laboratory Service Epidemiological Research Laboratory.

Dick, G. (1973) Register of cases of sub-acute sclerosing panencephalitis. *Br. med. J.*, iii, 359.

Doerr, R. & Schnabel, A. (1922) Herpes und Encephalitisvirus. *Schweiz. med. Wschr.*, 52, 325.

Dorfman, L. J. (1973) Cytomegalovirus encephalitis in adults. *Neurology*, 23, 136.

Editorial (1973) Herpes encephalitis. *Br. med. J.*, i, 582.

Flewett, T. M. & Hoult, J. G. (1958) Influenzal encephalopathy and post-influenzal encephalitis. *Lancet*, ii, 11.

Gajdusek, D. C. (1955) Encephalomyelitis infections in childhood. *Pediatrics, Springfield*, 16, 819.

Greenfield, J. G. (1950) Encephalitis and encephalomyelitis in England and Wales during the last decade. *Brain*, 73, 141.

Hartley, E. G. (1966) 'B' virus: herpes virus simiae. *Lancet*, i, 87.

Illis, L. S. & Gostling, J. V. T. (1972) In *Herpes Simplex Encephalitis*, p. 92. Bristol: Scientechnica.

General nature of viral encephalitis

Johnson, H. N. (1965) In *Viral and Rickettsial Infections of Man*, ed. Horsfall, F. L. & Tamm, I., p. 814. Philadelphia: Lippincott.

Juel-Jensen, B. E. & MacCallum, F. O. (1972) In *Herpes Simplex, Varicella and Zoster*, p. 113. London: Heinemann.

Lascelles, R. G., Longson, M., Johnson, P. J. & Chiang, A. (1973) Infectious mononucleosis presenting as acute cerebellar syndrome. *Lancet*, ii, 707.

Levaditi, C. & Harvier, P. (1920) Le virus de l'encéphalite léthargique. *C. r. Séanc. Soc. Biol., Paris*, 83, 354,

Liversedge, L. A., Longson, M. & MacCallum, F. O. (1972) Herpes encephalitis. *Br. med. J.*, iii, 527.

Muckenfuss, R. S., Armstrong, C. & McCordock, H. A. (1933) Encephalitis: Studies on experimental transmission. *Pub. Hlth Rep., Wash.*, 48, 1341.

Registrar General Statistical Review of England and Wales (annual). Part I. Tables, Medical. London: HMSO.

Remlinger, P. (1903) Le passage du virus rabique à travers les filtres. *Ann. Inst. Pasteur*, 17, 834.

Roos, R., Chou, S. M., Rogers, N. G., Basnight, M. & Gajdusek, D. C. (1972) Isolation of an Adenovirus 32 strain from human brain in a case of sub-acute encephalitis. *Proc. Soc. exp. Biol. Med.*, 139, 636.

Takagi, I. (1925) Etiology of encephalitis occurring epidemically in Japan. *Japan med. Wld*, 5, 147.

Termeulen, V., Muller, D., Kaciel, Y., Katz, Y. & Meyermann, R. (1972) Isolation of infectious measles virus in measles encephalitis. *Lancet*, ii, 1172.

World Health Organisation (1967) *Manual of the International Statistical Classification of Diseases, Injuries and Cause of Death*, vol. I, pp. 417–26. Geneva.

3

The Morphologist's Contribution to the Study of Viral Encephalitis

A. D. DAYAN
AND JUNE D. ALMEIDA

Morphological methods of study have contributed greatly to our knowledge of viral encephalitis, initially by the classical techniques of light microscopy, and subsequently by the more precise analyses permitted by immunofluorescence, autoradiography and electron microscopy. Light microscopy remains primarily a tool for diagnosis and the demonstration of patterns of disease. Immuno-fluorescence has become very important in the recognition of aetiological agents, as well as contributing information on the role of immunological reactions in viral encephalitis. Autoradiography has been principally a means for studying the cellular responses to infection of the brain (in animal systems). Lastly, electron microscopy has enabled classes of aetiological agents to be recognized, it has revealed modes of transport of viruses within the nervous system and, verging on the biochemical, it has shown something of the macromolecular events accompanying viral infection.

Various aspects of each of these methods are reviewed here, with particular reference to their value in diagnosis, and to some of the ways in which they have aided study of virally mediated tissue damage in the brain.

The normal nervous system is notorious for its complexity and the number and variety of artefacts apparent when it is studied by almost any means, effects which seem to be magnified when neural tissues are diseased. Some attention will be paid to morphological artefacts, as they have led to much unnecessary confusion and unrewarding speculation. The emphasis of this chapter has been placed deliberately on morphological methods, even though there are other techniques potentially far more valuable for the diagnosis of these particular neurological disorders. It is unfortunately true, however, that the first line of investigation of an atypical encephalitis is often by neuropathology, the correct diagnosis not having been suspected prior to autopsy and subsequent morbid anatomical examination. In addition, morphological methods have been revivified by the realization that the brain is too complex to be understood by any one approach, and that the findings of virological and biochemical techniques must be supported by visualization of the processes at work in the central nervous system.

GENERAL FEATURES OF VIRAL ENCEPHALITIS

Entry of a virus into the mature nervous system and its proliferation there may not produce any apparent change, or it may be accompanied by variable degrees of damage to parenchymal and stromal cells with accompanying inflammatory reaction and oedema. Such processes are identical to those found in any infected tissue or organ and they depend on the derangement of cell metabolism through direct growth of the virus, and the potentially harmful side-effects of immune mechanisms that the virus calls into action. Cells die and, because of the progressive active involvement of humoral and cell-mediated immune mechanisms, there is oedema and a reactive infiltration of acute and chronic inflammatory cells, including polymorphs, macrophages (derived both locally and from blood-borne precursors), lymphocytes and plasma cells. Blood vessels too may be damaged, either directly by the virus or by immunological reactions, and this, in turn, may cause secondary lesions and haemorrhages. Like any inflammatory disorder of the brain, virus encephalitis can cause damage indirectly through cerebral oedema, which in turn may result in extensive and even life-threatening lesions if vital areas are affected by intracranial hernias. A further indirect mechanism of damage that can be mediated by virus infection is the anoxia and impaired cerebral circulation secondary to *grand mal* epileptiform convulsions.

The consequences of viral infection of the developing nervous system are important because of the wide range of effects they can produce. These can range from discrete, readily apparent, anatomical defects or frankly pathological lesions (often not obviously inflammatory in nature) to more subtle clinical defects that may remain latent for years.

Although most viruses that cause encephalitis do so by affecting both neurones and glial cells, i.e. by causing some form of panencephalitis, more restricted forms do occur. Maximal damage may occur either to one specialized type of cell: 'polioencephalitis' if neurones are affected or 'leucoencephalitis' if damage is concentrated on the glial cells in white matter. The effects of a virus may also be limited to anatomically localized areas, e.g. particular nuclei, such as dorsal root or trigeminal ganglia, or restricted parts of the brain, such as the temporal lobe. The reasons for such effects are not known, but they may represent metabolic peculiarities of the cells concerned that render them particularly susceptible to infection by the virus concerned. Localization could also be dependent on cell-to-cell transfer of virus along a neural pathway, or to special anatomical vulnerability produced by the effects of intracranial herniation of the oedematous brain. There are several examples of viruses producing localized lesions in the CNS and some of the better known of these will now be considered.

Herpes zoster causes intense damage to one or two dorsal root ganglia, and perhaps less severe lesions in the corresponding segments of the cord, but does not normally extend further in the nervous system.

Herpes simplex has a marked propensity to produce its most

severe lesions in the so-called limbic lobe, i.e. the anatomically interconnected but physically separate series of grisea and neural pathways that consist of the olfactory areas of the brain, hippo-campus and adjacent medial temporal lobe structures, forniceal system, insula and possibly other associated nuclei. The most plausible explanation for this unique pattern of damage is the existence of anatomical pathways along which virus can spread preferentially between affected structures. This idea is not entirely satisfactory because other viruses that probably enter the CNS from the oropharynx or nose rarely produce similar lesions and, conversely, other systems of interconnected tracts and nuclei are almost never affected in this way.

Poliomyelitis is classically a disease of the motor neurones in the anterior horns and brain-stem, but it also causes extensive damage to other nuclei in the reticular formation, vestibular and red nuclei, cerebral motor cortex, etc. The lesions of rabies occur mainly in the mid-brain and medulla but the Negri bodies are found particularly in nerve cells in the dentate fascia of Ammon's horn.

Japanese B and western equine encephalitis show some pre-dilection for the basal ganglia, including the substantia nigra.

Unfortunately, no pattern of damage by itself is specific for a particular virus, but if the distribution of lesions is considered with other parameters, such as the clinical features of the disease, the presence and type of inclusion bodies and the nature of additional degenerative changes, then the range of putative aetiological agents becomes narrowed.

NAKED EYE EXAMINATION

Those who have dissected many bodies have at least learned to doubt, when others who are ignorant of anatomy and do not take the trouble to learn it are in no doubt at all.
Morgagni

In the majority of cases of virus encephalitis the external appearances of the brain are not diagnostic and may not even be suggestive of encephalitis, as there is usually only moderate oedema, and perhaps agonal haemorrhages and clouding of the pia–arachnoid by the associated leptomeningitis. Similarly, the cut surfaces of the brain and cord commonly show only slight oedema and perhaps a few punctate haemorrhages in areas of maximal damage. In late or recovered cases, no abnormality will be seen, except perhaps for greyness and slight shrinkage or unusual firmness in areas of diffuse scarring.

Deviations from such non-specific appearances arise if there has been severe damage concentrated in particular areas, e.g. the 'limbic lobe encephalitis' often caused by herpes simplex. In such cases, if the patient dies during the acute stages the affected areas are necrotic, softened and may be frankly haemorrhagic. Later they are gradually converted to tough, shrunken, yellow-grey scars with adherent, thickened leptomeninges. Superficially the external appearance of the base of such a brain with extensive damage to the orbital cortex and anteromedial parts of both temporal lobes may resemble the late effects of mechanical injury, as in a road traffic accident, but the latter does not usually produce such symmetrical or widespread lesions, nor are deeper areas affected.

Spinal nerve roots appear thin and grey if the cells of origin of their contained nerve fibres have been destroyed. In herpes zoster 2 or 3 consecutive posterior roots on one side will show this effect while in cases of poliomyelitis (or other viruses that affect anterior horn cells, e.g. certain members of the coxsackie group), many more scattered anterior roots are affected.

HISTOPATHOLOGICAL FEATURES

Although different viruses may have different target cells there are still sufficient features common to all forms of encephalitis to justify a synopsis of the lesions.

Microscopical appearances

In the early stage of infection the microscopical appearances are chromatolysis of neurones, readily visible in large cells, sometimes accompanied by the regenerative feature of an RNA-rich nuclear cap. Dying nerve cells follow the common pattern of pyknosis, prominent eosinophilia, shrinkage of the cell body and apical dendrite, apparent loss of the nucleus and eventually complete disappearance of the cell. The space left by the latter is quickly filled by oedema and reactive cell processes. Changes in glial cells are less readily followed because they are smaller and their peri-karya and processes can only be visualized by use of special stains. They, too, show shrinkage and loss of processes (e.g. clasmato-dendrosis of astrocytes) before disappearing. It is difficult to time these events in man, but they probably take 1 to 2 days at least, and possibly longer.

At the same time sequential, reactive inflammatory changes develop. First, local microglia become 'activated', as their processes shorten and their cell bodies and nuclei enlarge progressively until they are recognizable as macrophages, like those elsewhere in the body. In haematoxylin and eosin stained sections, microglia can best be visualized as elongated, rod-shaped nuclei, and these 'rod cells' cluster around dying cells to form glial 'knots' or 'stars'. Polymorphs and mononuclear cells accumulate to some extent in nearby blood vessels and may be found occasionally passing through their walls into the neuropil. After a few days there are definite perivascular cuffs of recognizable lymphocytes, perhaps some polymorphs, macrophages and other mononuclear cells. Some time later, perhaps from about one week onwards, these cuffs are several cells thick, they contain a few plasma cells and others with pyroninophilic cytoplasm, and occasional mitoses may be seen. Thin cuffs, mainly a scattering of lymphocytes, persist for many months, particularly in areas of severe damage, where there is also more marked parenchymatous infiltration. In the white matter macrophages laden with birefringent lipid debris are seen and these are termed 'compound granular corpuscles'. Lastly, scarring occurs by proliferation of fibrillary astrocytes, which can be seen in conventional sections as increased numbers of rounded, solitary or twinned vesicular nuclei, but they are better demonstrated by special stains. Similar scarring is seen in white matter, albeit modified to a rather slower tempo, particularly as the eventual disappearance of lipid-filled macrophages may take months. Further complications are produced by Wallerian degeneration of axons and their myelin sheaths that may extend centrifugally over considerable distances in lengthy tracts. There are also the effects of oedema, which can be seen both in the form of swollen oligodendroglia and in the chink-like intercellular spaces between fibres that become filled with faintly eosinophilic and PAS-positive fluid.

If damage is very severe, or if blood vessels are involved directly, there will be focal haemorrhages in the neuropil, and capillaries and other small vessels may show focal thromboses and frank fibrinoid necrosis of their walls. 'Necrotizing encephalitis', commonly due to herpes simplex, represents an extreme form of this process in which there is usually widespread fibrinoid necrosis of small blood vessels, haemorrhages and extensive destruction of the neural parenchyma. It is accompanied especially by acute polymorphonuclear cell infiltration and even by leucocytoclasis. At a later stage, this results in the appearance of recanalization and fragmentation and reduplication of basement membranes. Macrophages, too, become enmeshed in the outer coats of connective tissue and reticulin of blood vessels.

As the majority of cells in the CSF get there by passage through the walls of capillaries in the leptomeninges, choroid plexus and CNS, their numbers and types are a blurred reflection of what is happening to the neural parenchyma. Because of this, examination of the appearance and cell content of the cerebrospinal fluid is essential in the diagnosis of encephalitis, both intrinsically and to aid the exclusion of other, more remediable conditions. However, it must be remembered that, if there is a necrotizing inflammation, or if CSF is obtained very early in the course of encephalitis, there may only be a slight rise in the cell count, and these may be polymorphs, and even, erythrocytes rather than the more typical 'lymphocytes' found later on.

None of the appearances described so far is unique in isolation, but the overall pattern is virtually diagnostic of viral infection. In the vicinity of any destructive process in the brain there will be some inflammatory infiltration, with slight perivascular cuffing and prominence and activation of glia. However, under these circumstances there will not usually be multifocal or disseminated neuronal destruction and glial stars. Difficulties can arise if there is more severe damage, e.g. in the vicinity of an abscess or large infarct; this may be accompanied by some loss of nerve cells and even by the appearance of polymorphs, in which case it may be impossible in a small biopsy to decide between the various diagnostic possibilities on pathological grounds alone. Similar problems may arise in the examination of biopsy fragments obtained from a recent infarct, or from a patient whose brain has been damaged by severe hypotension, anoxia or hypoglycaemia. In the latter group of conditions, however, it is usual to find larger and more diffuse areas of necrosis of nerve cells, rather than the many very small foci seen in viral encephalitis, and for there to be much less inflammatory cellular infiltration and glial star formation than in the latter conditions.

The presence of a few mononuclear cells around blood vessels, as is common in the basal ganglia of elderly sufferers from cerebrovascular disease, should not be taken as evidence of encephalitis. Differential diagnosis from meningitis, either acute pyogenic or more chronic granulomatous forms, depends on recognition of the relative preponderance of inflammatory cells in the subarachnoid space and its direct extension into the perivascular Virchow–Robin spaces. The relatively little parenchymatous change that does occur is restricted to the superficial part of the cortex, or the areas adjacent to the ependyma in cases of ventriculitis.

Inclusion bodies

It is frequently and incorrectly presumed that viral encephalitides specifically are accompanied by the appearance of inclusion bodies in cells in the brain. Unfortunately, neurones are a rich source of many types of cytoplasmic and nuclear inclusions that have no association whatsoever with viral infection, e.g. Marinesco bodies in the nuclei of pigmented neurones of the substantia nigra, Bionchi bodies in the ependyma, cytoplasmic inclusions in thalamic neurones in aged animals and man, and Lewy bodies in pigmented nerve cells. Conversely, many viral encephalitides are either not associated at all with the formation of inclusion bodies, or with their appearance only as an ephemeral phase in the evolution of the disease.

When viral inclusion bodies are present, they are the sites either of synthesis or assembly of viral components, or of accumulations of virus-coded material, often psuedocrystalline masses of protein. As noted above, they should not themselves be regarded as diagnostic of viruses in general, and even more definitely not diagnostic of any specific agent, but, if accompanied by features of infection, their presence can be a comforting reassurance in the diagnosis of viral encephalitis.

In western European man, inclusion bodies may be found most often in acute herpes simplex encephalitis and in the temperate subacute sclerosing panencephalitis (SSPE) caused by a measles-like agent. In the tropics, their greatest value has been in the diagnosis of rabies, by the recognition of Negri or Lyssa bodies. They have been reported occasionally in other diseases in man, e.g. herpes zoster, and far more often in experimental infections of laboratory animals by many different viruses.

Both in herpes simplex and SSPE they tend to occur in the earlier, more active phases of the disease, or, in patients in whom damage is localized to particular areas of the brain, in which regions the infection appears most active. In later cases, or perhaps those with less florid lesions, inclusion bodies are less common and often cannot be found at all. This could have been anticipated from experiments in vitro in which the appearance of stainable inclusions has been dependent on at least 3 factors: the metabolic state of the cells, the multiplicity of infection; and the rate of viral proliferation.

The histochemical properties of inclusion bodies have not proved to be of as much value in their general differential diagnosis as has electron microscopy (see below).

Atypical encephalitis

In recent years three groups of infections of the CNS have been recognized which differ markedly from classical acute encephalitis, as described above. These are temperate or subacute encephalitis, infections in patients with defective immune responses, and the spongiform encephalopathies due to highly atypical 'slow viruses'. The fundamental importance of all these disorders lies in their similarities to other, often more common diseases, as yet of unknown aetiology and pathogenesis, and the need to be aware of the putative relationships so that appropriate investigations can be done.

The two principal temperate disorders are subacute sclerosing panencephalitis (SSPE) and progressive multifocal leucoencephalopathy (PML). The former evolves in young children over the course of several months and shows, as its name implies, subacute panencephalitis accompanied by dense gliotic scarring; there is often some selective demyelination too. The foci of neuronal and glial cell destruction, rod cell reaction and perivascular cuffing are not distributed uniformly through the neuraxis and pseudo-system lesions have been described. Thus, if specimens are examined from only a limited number of sites, an entirely erroneous diagnosis may be suggested. Large, Cowdry Type A, acidophilic inclusion bodies in neurones and glia are a striking feature of the disease but they may be present for only a limited period of time and even during that period may be very scarce. Their virtual absence from many of the cases examined led for some years to the separation as an independant disease of 'subacute sclerosing leucoencephalitis', a disorder dominated by gliotic scarring of white matter and a scanty inflammatory reaction. It is really one form, probably a later phase, of SSPE. The disease is due to persistent infection by a measles-like agent, the first direct evidence for which was obtained by electron microscope studies stimulated by the concurrence of inclusion bodies and inflammation.

Progressive multifocal leucoencephalopathy (PML) is an even rarer disease, occurring in an older age group and almost restricted to patients with a lymphoma, in which there are many small areas of demyelination associated with bizarrely distorted glial nuclei, some containing inclusion bodies, and minimal inflammatory reaction. Once again, the presence of inclusion bodies suggested a viral aetiology and this was proven subsequently by electron microscopy, and then by isolation of at least two viruses.

Encephalitis in patients with profound immunosuppression due to deliberate cytotoxic chemotherapy, widespread disease of lymphoid tissues or congenital defects in the formation of an immune response system, has been characterized by scattered necrosis of single nerve cells or small groups of cells, and the absence of perivascular inflammatory reaction, apart from some microglial–macrophage response, including the appearance of glial stars. Gliosis has been seen, too, as well as widespread necrosis in some cases, and sometimes inclusion bodies and distorted nuclei of glial and other cells. The overall appearance has been either of an indolent process, or of one modified by the lack of host response towards the occurrence of extensive necrosis without acute inflammation, features that may be contrasted with the histological consequences of the normal patient's vigorous response. The diagnostic points in the very heterogenous immunosuppressed group, against which to judge further possible instances, comprise at least some features of an inflammatory response, even if only in terms of macrophage activation, accompanied by necrosis or other disturbance of neuronal and glial morphology. In some cases, there have been demyelination, inclusion bodies and even extensive areas of gliosis.

SSPE is the only one of these conditions in which there is no *a priori* reason to anticipate defective immunity. It is also the only one of these conditions that shows well-marked cellular reaction in the form of perivascular cuffs of lymphocytes, plasma and other pyroninophilic cells, presumptive 'immunoblasts'.

Based on the histopathological findings, it is an interesting exercise to assess the morphological evidence that other diseases of the CNS might be due to temperate viral infections. Multiple sclerosis seems to be a particularly strong candidate, and so must be parkinsonism of the so-called 'post-encephalitic' type. The inflammatory type of neurological disorder occasionally associated with malabsorption syndromes also fits these criteria, as do the neurological complications of Behcet's syndrome, certain forms of carcinomatous neuromyopathy and transverse myelitis. On the other hand, the lack of any of the previously described features affords some weak evidence against a direct viral aetiology of such disorders as post-vaccinal and post-exanthematous demyelination, Devic's neuromyelitis optica, typical cases of subacute myelo-opticoneuritis (SMON), mainly found in Japan, and amyotrophic lateral sclerosis.

The spongiform encephalopathies, represented in man by Jakob–Creutzfeldt disease and kuru, and in animals by scrapie in sheep and the transmissible encephalopathy of mink, comprise a unique group. All of them have now been shown to be transmissible by cell-free filtrates, either to the original host species or, in the instance of the human diseases, to chimpanzees and other primates. They stand out by their common features of a genetic background, silent period of incubation for years, lack of any apparent inflammatory or immunological response, diverse properties of their causal agents and, positively, by their unique pathological combination of neuronal loss, often of system type, intense glial proliferation and spongy intra- and intercellular vacuolation. Many cases also show interstitial amyloid-like plaques somewhere in the brain. Their remarkable histological characteristics, together with the fact that it has so far proved impossible to characterize or recover the aetiological agents, means that final diagnostic proof of a member of the group depends entirely on light microscope appearances. Despite much fruitless speculation, no other diseases have yet been found that even come near to this combination of features, so the group remains confined to four conditions. In spite of this there have been potential candidates, albeit increasingly unlikely ones, but large numbers of animals have failed to manifest illnesses even after experimental inoculation for periods of many years. These candidates have included the parkinsonism–dementia complex found in Guam and other communities in Asia, motor neurone disease, supranuclear ophthalmoplegia etc. In this context it is interesting that hypertrophy and perhaps hyperplasia of astrocytes have been illustrated in the brain after a variety of immunization procedures in experimental animals. So far these observations remain as striking experiments and their relevance to diseases of man has still to be determined.

ELECTRON MICROSCOPY

The analytical power of electron microscopy as applied to viral encephalitis has lain in its ability to demonstrate directly presumed aetiological agents; to illustrate likely pathogenetic mechanisms of cell and tissue damage and repair; and to reveal some of the macromolecular biochemical processes involved in these reactions.

So far, detection of virions and their characterization at least to group level have been among the most striking successes of electron microscopy in neuropathology. It has been a valuable aid in diagnosis, sometimes even during life. Using this method to study material from acute necrotizing encephalitis it has been possible to implicate herpesvirus as the aetiological agent, to confirm adenovirus infections and to detect various features of rabies in the brain. However, it has been from the temperate disorders that the most valuable results have come. Without the revelation by electron microscopy of paramyxovirus-like tubules in SSPE and polyoma-like virions in PML, it would be unlikely even today that virologists would have applied the effort necessary to isolate these agents. One of the strengths of electron microscopy is that, while correctly processed tissue yields the best results, it is still possible to examine material with a far from satisfactory history. Many virions will survive the slowest autopsy, and even stained light microscope sections and museum specimens can be reprocessed successfully for thin sectioning.

Up to this point the only electron microscope technique that has been considered is that of thin section transmission microscopy. A major advantage of this method is that tissue architecture is maintained and resolution is such that it is possible to visualize not only complete virus but also viral components. However, preparation of tissue for thin sectioning requires extremely small

44

pieces of tissue, about 1 mm face which may cause serious difficulties of sampling. In order to avoid this situation it is sometimes possible to employ the electron microscope technique of negative staining for the examination of brain tissue that may contain virus. Negative staining does not preserve tissue structure but, because it is carried out on a brain homogenate, there is very little sampling effect. In practice it is done by making a 10% suspension of brain tissue in normal saline and then centrifuging at an intermediate speed, e.g. 20 minutes at 10 000 rpm, the supernatant being used for negative staining. The very real advantages of this technique are those already mentioned, namely that there is little or no sampling effect, and also that if virus particles can be seen, then the technique will also reveal their substructure (Plate I/1/2, Plate II). The value of the latter is that it is the basis for placing the agent in its correct morphological category. At an even simpler level the presence of substructure means that it is possible to state definitively that the structure is a virus, something that it is not always possible to do with material prepared by thin sectioning, as brain tissue contains so many virus-like objects. However, negative staining will only be successful if virus particles are present in concentrations of approx. 10^6 particles/ml of brain suspension. Below this level the 'signal to noise' ratio is such that there is little hope of seeing and recognizing a virus.

It is sometimes possible to improve this situation by adding antiserum against the suspected virus to the brain suspension. If virus is present, it will be clumped by the antibody and will then become much more prominent on the microscope grid. This is particularly useful when the virus that is being sought has little distinctive morphology, e.g. picornaviruses and togaviruses. In addition, negative staining of brain suspension can sometimes yield additional, unsuspected information. In a recent example, brain material was received from a suspected case of SSPE and thin section studies revealed myxovirus-type tubules within neurones. Negative staining also revealed myxovirus-type tubules showing the typical herring bone arrangement of the nucleoprotein. In addition, it was found that the majority of these tubules were covered by what appeared to be antibody molecules even though, in this case, no antiserum had been added to the preparation. The explanation was almost certainly that the brain tissue contained residual amounts of blood and that on homogenization there was sufficient antibody present to attach to the virus component. This morphological result has shown how quickly and with how little apparent contamination virus can be coated with antibody and, by extrapolation, inactivated during a simple step, such as preparation of a homogenate. In the case of SSPE it is of additional interest as there is good reason to suspect that there is an immune aspect to this abnormal infection with measles virus, and the observation finding has confirmed the presence within an SSPE-affected brain both of virus and antibody.

Unfortunately, in the case of neuropathological specimens, the technique of negative staining has several drawbacks. As already stated, the virus must be present in sufficient quantity to make visualization possible. There is no means of correlating virus with tissue architecture, as the technique is carried out on a homogenate. Previously fixed specimens cannot be used for negative staining, as the tissue must be fresh. The latter is possibly the greatest drawback of the technique, as it is often only after either light microscope or thin section electron microscope examination that it is realized that negative staining would have been important. Thin section electron microscopy often reveals large numbers of small round particles that *could* be virus in the CNS. However, the CNS contains many small round structures that are entirely normal, and without the definitive substructural evidence of negative staining it is impossible to substantiate many of these results. There is, therefore, a very good case to be made for freezing at −20°C or lower, small pieces of biopsy or autopsy tissue from cases that could, even remotely, be of viral origin.

The discussion of negative staining has emphasized the point that thin sectioned neuropathological material, in particular, suffers from the presence of numerous unidentifiable structures. Under some circumstances nerve arborizations, microtubules, neurofilaments and nuclear pores can all appear virus-like. Some of these structures are sufficiently virus-like to make it impossible to distinguish them on the basis of thin section evidence alone. It must be reiterated, therefore, that in order to characterize a virus with certainty it is necessary to study substructure by means of the negative staining technique. By this method virus morphology can be defined with such precision, that only rarely will an experienced observer remain in doubt about the significance of his findings.

IMMUNOFLUORESCENCE

The development of immunofluorescence techniques by Coons and his colleagues has permitted very detailed and wide ranging studies of the processes involved in viral infection of the nervous system and of the host's reponses. Almost for the first time the morbid anatomist as morphologist has been able to dissect and assess dynamically modes of infection, viral transport and replication, as well as certain features of the immune response.

The technique usually requires preservation of small blocks of tissues by snap freezing at a low temperature and the cutting of cryostat sections. In this way histological detail is retained and viral and other antigens are not denatured. Sections are exposed to an antibody against the antigen of interest, either already coupled to a fluorescent dye ('direct' immunofluorescence), or they are treated with an intermediate layer of non-fluorescent antiserum and then exposed to a further solution of a fluorescent-labelled antibody against the intermediate antiserum (the indirect or 'sandwich' technique). When examined by microscopy with suitable blue light or ultra-violet illumination, fluorescent areas represent the sites of the chosen antigen, and they can be seen at the same time as full histological detail. The principal difficulties of immunofluorescence are ensuring that tissue is preserved suitably (if specimens from suspected cases are saved for electron microscopy, then additional blocks should also be kept for immunofluorescence), and the preparation and standardization of potent, specific antisera.

Viral antigens and viral behaviour

The portals of entry of viruses into the CNS under natural conditions, as demonstrated by immunofluorescence and other means, may be via the conjunctiva, the nose and oropharynx, various levels of the gastrointestinal tract (notably the large and perhaps the small intestine), and via the blood stream if infection is produced by a biting insect or trauma. In the majority of instances there is a phase of local replication of virus at the site of entry, followed by generalized viraemia before the agent penetrates into the nervous system. The subsequent route of entry then may be via sites of lower efficiency of the 'blood–brain barrier', or by the several mechanisms that can transport particulate structures across blood vessel walls, e.g. pinocytosis, penetration through intercellular gaps, carriage in white cells that undergo diapedesis etc. The role of infected leucocytes or macrophages in the dissemination of infection probably depends on the nature of the virus and on physiological factors that influence the pinocytotic and virucidal activities of the cells. Certainly, they may help to spread infection as much as to combat it. One aspect of this may be the demonstration in encephalitis of viral antigens both in white cells and in the CSF, as well as in the cells of the perivascular cuffs of reactive inflammatory infiltration. In rabies, herpes simplex and herpes zoster clear evidence has been provided by the immunofluorescent demonstration of viral antigens that infection may track directly along peripheral nerve axis cylinders and their Schwann cell sheaths to gain access to the brain or cord. A spurious appearance of localized neural transport to the brain or cord can occur if neurones in a restricted anatomical region have been stimulated from outside to a particularly high level of activity. Local vascular permeability will then be accentuated and a generalized viraemia may have its first or most severe effect at that site, thus mimicking neural carriage of virus.

Immunofluorescence has shown that, once virus is in the brain, viral proliferation occurs in various types of cells. Parenthetically, it should be noted that identification of cell types in the CNS is extremely difficult, even if the histologist has the aid of all his classical staining methods. It is no wonder that naive attempts to

PLATE I

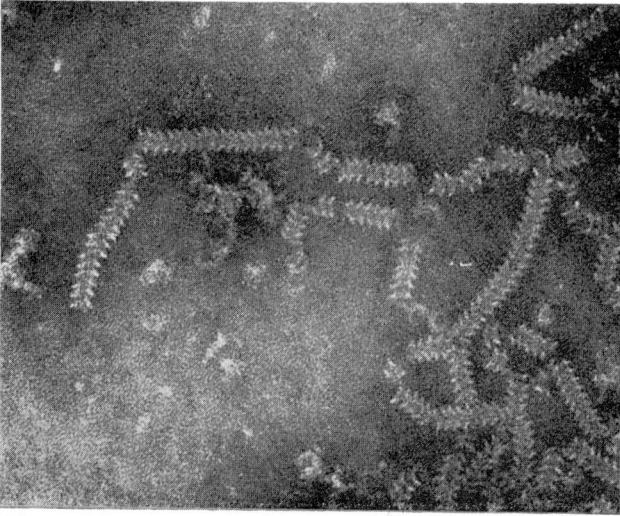

Fig. 1. Negatively stained ribonucleic core of the measles virus, showing the characteristic helical structure. The molecular architecture displayed so clearly can be of great help in detection, preliminary classification and proof of the viral aetiology of a suspected viral encephalitis.

× 115 500

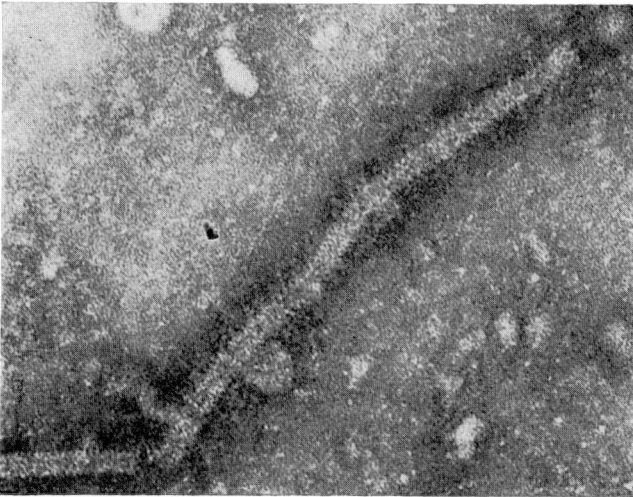

Fig. 2. A similar preparation from the brain of the patient suffering from subacute sclerosing panencephalitis, described in the text. The appearance of the helix has been partly obscured by attached antibody molecules.

× 115 500

PLATE II

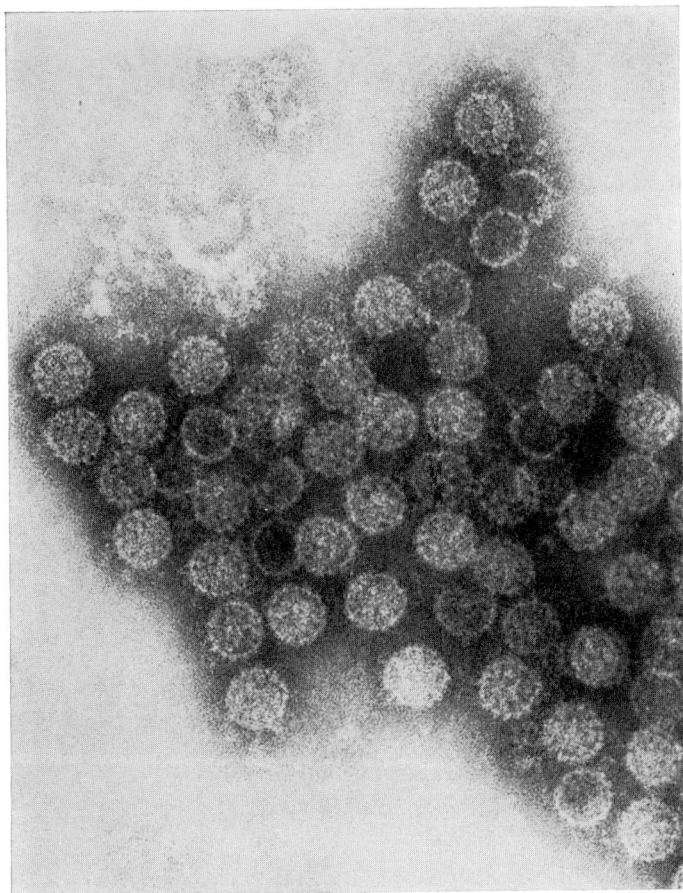

Fig. 1. Empty and full particles of Jakob–Creutzfeldt virus from a patient suffering from progressive multifocal leukoencephalopathy. Detail of capsomere arrangement and number is visible, which, together with the size and shape of the virus, is of great help in identification and classification.

× 115 500

identify cells in thin, cryostat sections, with their numerous artefacts and generally unusual appearances, have led to such confusion. In spite of this it has been possible to trace the spread of
antigens through cell processes along nerve tracts or systems. At
least in temperate encephalitides, it is common to find restricted
foci of viral antigen, perhaps groups of 100 or fewer cells, with
demonstrable antigen in their processes, separated by several
millimetres of apparently normal brain. This phenomenon may
be an example of local direct cell to cell spread of infection
through the neuropil, a process encouraged, or so it is presumed,
by shielding of intracellular virus from the host's immune defences.
This may be so but it depends on the nature and time of appearance of viral or other neo-antigens on the cell surface, and the
immune responses to them, topics which still await examination in
the practical complexities of the nervous system.

Still using immunofluorescence, cellular sites of synthesis of
viral components have been studied in man and in animals,
and differences have been revealed between the excessive sim-
plicity of homogenous tissue cultures in vitro and the considerable
heterogeneity of real life. The demonstration in SSPE that the
commonest site of antigen was intranuclear, as opposed to the
intracytoplasmic virus factories of more typical measles infections,
was important in suggesting the occurrence of a 'defective' infection in that disease.

Immunofluorescence has considerable value for diagnosis, both
in the clinical situation because of its speed, and as a research tool
in unusual cases, where it need not require large amounts of tissue
and complex facilities for viral isolation or serology—only a
few suitable sections and a small amount of antiserum. Its dis-
advantages are the need to have the appropriate antiserum and
the risk of artefact. The latter may be due to non-specificity of
antiserum and to artefactual positives, both topics of infinite
appeal to the technologist. The nervous system seems particularly
prone to artefactual staining as reactive cells, especially astrocytes,
easily pick up over-concentrated reagents. The well-known artefactual 'dark cell' should be another constant cause of concern,
because it readily takes up almost any antiserum to which it is

exposed. These potential errors can only be avoided by frequently testing the specificity of antisera, including use of known infected neural tissue, and asking whether the morphology of every fluorescent cell or other structure is that of a known CNS constituent (and not a 'dark' or 'dying' cell), and whether it appears reasonable from other evidence that it should contain virus. For example, the use of over-concentrated antisera often results in fluorescence restricted just to fibrillary astrocytes which otherwise appear entirely normal. Consecutive or simultaneous transmitted light phase contrast examination of immunofluorescent sections is invaluable. Attempts have occasionally been made to explain failure to demonstrate viral antigens by suggesting that they might be covered or 'masked' by a layer of autologous antibody. If these sections are treated in such a way as to dissociate the presumed antigen–antibody complexes, staining may be produced by an appropriate viral antiserum. Although such a mechanism is theoretically feasible, it is highly unlikely in practice that host antibody would conceal completely all the viral antigens, and post-dissociation staining is far more likely to be an artefact.

There is a paramount need in the field of neuropathology for the usual controls of immunofluorescence, as well as comparison with normal brain treated in the same way, and morphological acceptability of the eventual fluorescent image.

As judged by published evidence, both snap-frozen cryostat sections and cold alcohol fixed (Saint-Marie technique) paraffin-embedded material are equally liable to these artefacts. As freezing is so much easier, and as the cytological detail visible in cryostat sections can approach that of paraffin-embedded material, the former appears to be the better method of preservation for routine purposes.

Immunological processes
As in many other aspects of medicine, immunofluorescent techniques have had a prime role in demonstration of the site and nature of the local humoral immune response to infection of the nervous system. The perivascular cuffs initially include IgM-containing cells, which are succeeded after a few days by a pre-

ponderance of IgG-containing plasma cells and pyroninophilic immunocytes. This switch mirrors the conventional change in antibody type in a primary immune response. Little attempt appears to have been made to employ specific anti-κ or anti-λ antisera to demonstrate the clones of antibody producing cells known to occur in chronic infections. The involvement of cell-mediated immunity is more difficult to demonstrate by immuno-fluorescence, but it might be possible by careful use of fluorescent T-cell marker sera under conditions suitable for demonstration of surface antigens.

A relatively neglected aspect from the standpoint of immuno-fluorescence is study of the existence and mechanisms of immuno-logical damage to infected tissues. Thus, either by restaining, or better by use of a double antibody method with labels that fluoresce at different wave-lengths, it may be possible to demon-strate binding of IgM or IgG and the β_1c (C'3) component of com-plement to the same cell. Such evidence provides strong circum-stantial support for the possibility of direct antibody-mediated cytotoxicity (Type II) reaction. In some forms of encephalitis, e.g. herpes simplex, as well as in some cases of acute para-infectious demyelination, fibrinoid necrosis of small blood vessels in the brain may be seen. The likelihood of immune complex deposition leading to a Type III reaction under these circumstances has been greatly strengthened by immunofluorescent demonstration of bound IgG and β_1c in vessel walls, and sometimes even of viral antigen there.

Putative Type III reactions and circulating immune complexes of antibody and viral antigen have recently been demonstrated in human and experimental encephalitides, with dissemination of viral antigen (and possibly intact viable virus) throughout the body. Proof of the occurrence of such processes and their demon-stration have become tools for basic immunological research into the causes and mechanisms of immune complex formation, and their vascular and visceral effects. They have also led to specula-tions about the efficacy of immunological responses in determining the course of an infection: at least in so far as the production of complexes depends on genotype as well as the nature and dose of antigen. In man, therefore, demonstration of complexes (easiest for the morphologist in the kidney), or of widespread visceral deposits of virus in cells of the reticulo-endothelial system, may be indirect evidence of quantitative variation in immune response and of the systemic effects of a particular genetic constitution.

AUTORADIOGRAPHY

The methods of radio-labelling cells, e.g. with ^{3}H-thymidine etc., to indicate their origins, or to demonstrate the synthesis of DNA, have been of value experimentally in showing how inflammatory cellular infiltration in brain is largely derived from haematogenous cells. Smaller particulate or soluble markers (labelled proteins and Thorotrast) have aided demonstration of the permeability mechanisms involved in viral infection and consequent cerebral oedema. These techniques are of very limited applicability to man because of the ethical and practical difficulties of administration of radio-isotopes to patients.

A further technique potentially of extreme value in elucidating the agents responsible for certain hitherto obscure inflammatory conditions, is autoradiographic demonstration in host cells of nucleic acids homologous with nucleic acid sequences in particular viruses. In other tissues, these sequences have been found in the nuclei of cells in which no other features of infection were apparent, e.g. the Epstein-Barr virus in cells of Burkitt's lymphoma. A start has been made in the employment of this method to neurological diseases by reports of the finding of herpes simplex DNA in trigeminal ganglion cells from cases of trigeminal neuralgia. Its future value should be considerable, particularly as it does not necessarily require viral isolation from diseased tissues, something which may be extremely difficult in encephalitis.

CONCLUSIONS AND SPECULATIONS

The history of pathology in general and of neuropathology in particular has been one of increasing precision and refinement.

Observations were made originally with the naked eye, then came an era of light microscopy, to be followed by present development of the ultra-violet and electron microscopes. Each time a basic technical advance has been made, the simple science of morphological observation has obtained a fresh lease of life. The fruitful days of Virchow and Cajal made neuropathology an acceptable science, and the fine anatomy of the brain an exact study. Hopefully, we are approaching a new golden age, when the use of tools such as the electron microscope will advance the morphological study of neural cells to demonstration of the macromolecular processes being carried on in them. The morphologist has every reason to expect that his unique ability to dissect regional, cytological and even subcellular specialization will be in increasing demand, particularly as newer computer techniques for quantitative histology 'substitute brass for brain in the great labour of calculating'.

To predict future advances in any defined topic can never be better than pious speculation, but there seems a good chance of meeting the following suggestions in a reasonable time:

Light microscopy
Once it is accepted that viral infection does not lead inevitably to cell death, the inescapable question arises of how such cells are affected? Do they become stunted, are their unique arborizations of processes lost, and is there any persisting abnormality of metabolism? Provided these cells can be identified, perhaps by the presence of inclusion bodies or immunofluorescent demonstration of viral antigens, then the morphological approach affords a unique opportunity to examine the wealth and connectivity of processes by Golgi-type staining, and aspects of metabolism by quantitative interference microscopy, cytochemistry and autoradiography. Even simple measurement of cellular, nuclear or nucleolar size could be of importance. Classical histochemistry has contributed little to the study of encephalitis so far, with the exception of providing information on the type of nucleic acid present in inclusion bodies, but its opportunity to be of value could come in quantitative measures of functional parameters.

Immunofluorescence

Quantitation of antigens is possible here, too, so it should be possible to make far more detailed examinations of the manner and timing of viral reproduction and assembly, as well as of changes in host cell components. The role of the host's immune reactions requires further analysis in relation to the proximate or final causes of tissue damage and inflammatory reactions.

All these methods are as applicable to specimens obtained from man as to material from experimental infections. The importance of this lies in the present lack of animal models of many of the temperate and other atypical viral diseases of man.

Autoradiography

The most immediate objective of autoradiography ought to be application of the radioactive DNA technique for demonstration of homologues of viral DNA to such problem diseases as multiple sclerosis and cerebral tumours.

Isotope techniques afford an additional means of measuring aspects of cellular metabolism, e.g. protein or lipid synthesis, which ought to be examined in chronically infected neurones and glia.

Electron microscopy

Neural tissue has presented many problems to the electron microscopist. Perhaps the most important is that presented by the size of many neural cells. Processes up to several micrometres long are common and extensions of many centimetres do occur. The limited block size possible in the electron microscope means that it is almost impossible to obtain continuity over these distances, and consequently it is difficult to build up an integral image at the electron microscope level. Increasing knowledge of the normal fine structural appearances of the brain makes it possible to recognize at a subcellular level the changes induced by pathological processes. The possibility of visualizing virus particles and components within cells of the CNS alone makes it an extremely powerful tool in the study of diseases of known or suspected viral origin. Additional electron microscope techniques, such as negative staining and immune electron microscopy, will almost certainly widen the applicability of this instrument in subsequent years.

Finally, although morphological observation is the simplest of the techniques that might be applied to the study of disease processes in the central nervous system, it must also be remembered that one clear picture is worth a thousand words.

FURTHER READING

Melnick, J. L. (1974) Slow viruses. *Prog. Med. Virol.*, **18.**

Nathanson, N. & Cole, G. A. (1970) Immunosuppression and viral encephalitis. *Adv. viral Res.*, **16,** 397.

Van Bogaert, L., Radermecker, J., Hozay, J. & Lowenthal, A. (1961) *Encephalitides*. Amsterdam: Elsevier.

4

Laboratory Diagnosis of Viral Encephalitis

J. V. T. GOSTLING

The commonest cause of severe sporadic acute encephalitis is herpes simplex virus and the major part of this chapter is devoted to the investigation of this condition. Every aspect has been the subject of much attention in recent publications, but first other diseases will be reviewed.

At the Congress of Scandinavian neurologists in 1972 Ivar Helle, talking about newer diagnostic and therapeutic methods, complained that there was not much new in the literature about acute types of encephalitis as compared with the abundant work on 'slow virus'. He divides acute types prevalent in Scandinavia into 'primary' with damage of CNS cells by virus and 'para-infectious' associated with an immunological reaction.

In his primary group the aetiological agents which he includes are enteroviruses, *Herpesvirus hominis*, arboviruses and the virus of mononucleosis and mumps; these are joined with qualifying question marks by adenoviruses and influenza viruses. The agents of parainfectious encephalitis listed are rubella, varicella and vaccinia. Measles appears in both lists.

Helle is realistically discouraging about diagnostic help from the laboratory. The diagnosis will be primarily clinical, substantiated by EEG. Examination of cerebrospinal fluid is not helpful. Some-how encephalitis must be differentiated from sepsis, intoxication, vascular catastrophes, trauma and 'expansive processes'. Definite aetiological diagnosis will be made by methods which apply equally to viral meningitis and will be achieved when the patient has recovered.

Also in 1972 a Symposium on Clinical Neurology contained an article by Miller and Harter on 'Acute viral encephalitis'. Though citing more than 80 references these authors confine themselves to infections caused by arboviruses or *Herpesvirus hominis* as being the main agents responsible respectively for epidemic and sporadic encephalitis in the United States. They remark on the rarity of arbovirus isolation from blood or cerebrospinal fluid and state that diagnosis depends on antibody titrations in recovered patients.

A less recent but more useful review was published in 1967 by Kennedy and Wanglee from the Children's Hospital of Philadelphia. They give some figures for the frequency of encephalitis as a complication of the commoner virus infections.

Kennedy and Wanglee list the infections shown in Table 4 under the heading 'post-infectious encephalitis'. They clearly include not only those illnesses called by Helle (1972) 'para-infectious' but some of those which he would call 'primary'.

Kennedy and Wanglee make two points which, though not

TABLE 4

POST-INFECTIOUS ENCEPHALITIS

Infection	Incidence of encephalitis	Mortality
Vaccinia	1 per 10^3 (Europe)	Not stated
	1 per 5×10^5 (USA)	Not stated
Measles	60–65 per 10^5	12%
Varicella	3 per 10^3	28%
Mumps	5–100 per 10^3*	1% (meningoencephalitic form)
		20% (less frequent encephalitic form)
Rubella	'Infrequent'	'High'

Data from Kennedy and Wanglee (1972).
* From Henle and Enders (1965).

57

original, deserve emphasis. First that 'encephalitis' is a term often loosely applied to unexplained febrile encephalopathy in which other possible causes for the symptoms have been ruled out. Second that a cellular response in the cerebrospinal fluid does not occur in at least a third of cases of encephalitis, and does occur quite often in infectious disease without signs or symptoms referable to the CNS.

McKendrick, in a letter to the *Lancet* in 1968, said that the relative frequency of the various causes of encephalitis would depend upon the sort of hospital in which the observer worked. He, writing from an infectious disease unit in north London, found the most common association was with measles or chicken-pox; but even more common were the cases he called 'primary encephalitis', in which there was no indication as to what the aetiological agent might be. He stated that diagnosis was difficult but, apart from considering brain biopsy a useful aid in severe cases, he mentions no laboratory procedures.

CLINICAL PATHOLOGY

Having emphasized that the laboratory can give little help to the clinician in establishing that the patient has inflammation of the brain substance, regardless of its aetiology and having noted that recent clinical contributors to the literature are aware of the laboratory's limitations in this respect, one may consider the clinical pathology of encephalitis.

The peripheral blood
The cellular and chemical constituents of the blood are unaffected by virus encephalitis; secondary bacterial infection will cause characteristic changes in the absolute and relative numbers of the white cells; dehydration may affect the levels of soluble constituents. The encephalitis itself may be a complication in a patient with an underlying pathological or iatrogenic abnormality of the blood.

The cerebrospinal fluid

The writer believes that cerebrospinal fluid (CSF) should be obtained by lumbar puncture in all suspected cases of encephalitis. There are dissenters from this belief. I recall a meeting at the Children's Hospital of Philadelphia to decide upon a regimen for the initial management of children admitted with suspected encephalitis. The incidence of lead poisoning in Philadelphia was high at that time. The senior resident physician had recently seen a sudden death in a child with lead encephalopathy caused by 'coning' of brain substance in the foramen magnum when CSF under high pressure was released by lumbar puncture: he was reluctant to agree that lumbar CSF should be obtained in all cases. A visiting Australian paediatrician, who had not encountered lead poisoning, thought that lumbar puncture was indispensable; and the paediatric neurologist, though well aware of lead encephalopathy, said that lumbar puncture must be done despite the slight risk.

Though we have seen in earlier paragraphs that clinicians expect little positive help from examination of the CSF in confirmation of a diagnosis of encephalitis, it will help to exclude such differential diagnoses as bacterial meningitis and intracranial haemorrhage (Bower 1969).

Findings which have been reported in encephalitis include:

A few lymphocytes, in no case more than 20/mm³ in 14 of 23 cases; and a syphilitic type of Lange curve (with negative Wassermann reaction) in 17 of 21 cases of encephalitis lethargica in children. CSF pressure was raised in some of these cases: sugar was present in all (Findlay & Shiskin 1921).

16 cells (15 lymphocytes) with normal chemistry, in a case of Coxsackie B2 encephalitis (Bower 1969).

500 to 3000 cells, at first mostly polymorphonuclear but later mostly lymphocytes, in a cloudy fluid with raised protein and normal sugar, under increased pressure in cases of eastern equine encephalitis (Miller & Harter 1972).

Up to 200 cells, predominantly mononuclear in fluid under normal pressure, in western equine encephalitis (Miller & Harter 1972).

A normal fluid or a moderate pleocytosis in viral or presumed viral encephalitides (Scott 1969).

CSF collected at the earliest opportunity is valuable, too, for attempts to make an aetiological diagnosis by virus isolation and by comparison with later specimens, for the detection of an increased amount of antibody to a particular virus.

The clinical pathology of acute necrotizing encephalitis due to herpes simplex virus will be considered later.

From our laboratory, which receives specimens by post, rail and van collection from several parts of the southern counties, one must rely on clinical comments made on request forms by colleagues. From this remote viewpoint it appears that mumps is the laboratory diagnosis most commonly associated with a clinical diagnosis of encephalitis.

Tables 5 to 7 show details of patients with mumps confirmed in the laboratory by virus isolation or, more commonly, by finding a rising titre of complement-fixing antibody.

TABLE 5

SYMPTOMS IN 79 PATIENTS WITH MUMPS
CONFIRMED BY LABORATORY DIAGNOSIS

Symptom	No. of patients
Meningitis	28
Meningoencephalitis	7
Encephalitis	3
Convulsions	4
No CNS involvement	37

TABLE 6

AGE AND SEX DISTRIBUTION OF
42 PATIENTS WITH CNS INVOLVEMENT

Age	Male	Female
Less than 11 years	26	9
Aged 12–20	—	—
More than 21 years	4	3

TABLE 7

TEST BY WHICH DIAGNOSIS WAS MADE
IN 79 PATIENTS

Test	No. of patients
Virus isolation only	5 (2 CSF; 3 T/S)
Rising CF antibody titre versus virus and/or soluble mumps antigen	71
Virus isolation and rising antibody titre	3 (CSF)

Of course the proportion of cases with central nervous system involvement shown in these tables is much higher than the true figure for all cases of mumps. The reason for this is that in uncomplicated mumps doctors are unlikely to send specimens to us. Estimates of the true percentage of mumps cases with involvement of the CNS range from 0·5 to 10%.

I think that the small number of patients probably accounts for absence of older children and adolescents—no meningitis or encephalitis between 11 and 21 years of age. But the preponderance of boys over girls is well known and is said by Henle and Enders (1965) to be up to five-fold.

The ratio of cases in which the doctor thought there was some brain involvement to those with meningitis only—about 1 to 2—is higher than in our larger series of laboratory-confirmed enterovirus infections.

In this group, Table 8 which does not incidentally include any patients infected with polioviruses, the cases with clinical evidence of encephalitis are much less numerous than those with meningitis only.

In the laboratory during the period covered by Tables 5–7 we received specimens from 36 patients with measles confirmed serologically: three were thought clinically to have encephalitis. Of 35 cases of varicella–zoster infection confirmed in the laboratory in the same period, one, a 4-year-old girl, had encephalitis.

The large group of encephalitides of unknown aetiology—

TABLE 8

SYMPTOMS IN 254 PATIENTS WITH ENTEROVIRUS
INFECTION CONFIRMED BY LABORATORY DIAGNOSIS

Symptom	*No. of patients*	
Meningitis	78	
Encephalitis	4	(1 ECHO 3, CSF; 1 Coxsackie A9, CSF; 1 Coxsackie B3, faeces; 1 rising CF titre to Coxsackie B5)
Convulsions	3	(1 ECHO 7, CSF; 1 Coxsackie B4, faeces; 1 rising CF titre to Coxsackie B5)
No CNS involvement	169	

nearly half the cases in McKendrick's experience—include, apart from those cases resembling one of the more common viral encephalitides in which the laboratory fails to identify the agent, some clinically distinguishable entities.

One of these is encephalitis lethargica. This condition is not seen nowadays, though some doctors working in mental hospitals claim to see post-encephalitic parkinsonism in patients too young to have been infected before 1927. I have already referred to studies of the cerebrospinal fluid in children with this condition made by Findlay and Shiskin in 1920. The historical introduction to their paper quotes reports of outbreaks of similar illnesses in various parts of Europe in 1712, 1768, 1785, 1800, 1802 and 1890. So perhaps encephalitis lethargica may return and give us a chance to look for the aetiological agent causing it.

BENIGN MYALGIC ENCEPHALOMYELITIS

In the review of 14 outbreaks of illness with the characteristics of this disease which Acheson published in 1959, using the synonyms 'Iceland disease' and 'epidemic neuromyasthenia', he noted that laboratory findings were mostly negative. In only 14 patients of 194 subjected to lumbar puncture did the CSF contain more than

5 lymphocytes/mm³; in only 11 was the protein concentration more than 40 mg/100 ml. Despite intensive attempts to isolate viruses in several of the outbreaks, the only finding was poliovirus 3 in the faeces of one patient who did not develop antibody to that agent. Nothing distinctive was found on EEG, but electromyography of affected muscles showed grouping of action potentials between regular intervals of complete inactivity, giving rise to a tremulous contraction at a frequency of 5 to 10 per second. These changes were reported in the Royal Free outbreak by Richardson (1956), in Ramsay's series (1957) and in Galpine and Brady's (1957) Coventry cases.

More than 10 years after Acheson's review there was a small outbreak of publications on this subject. Those by psychiatrists (McEvedy & Beard 1970), attributing the symptoms to something in the minds of the patients and their doctors, have no relevance to the laboratory diagnosis of encephalitis. A paper by Innes (1970) from Edinburgh is interesting to a laboratory reader, in that the 4 patients he describes with an illness clinically resembling benign myalgic encephalomyelitis all had evidence of current or recent enterovirus infection; and this despite the fact that none of them were investigated until they had been unwell for 3 months or more. Innes concluded that, unless his patients were cases of motor neurone disease, they must be examples of the condition reviewed by Acheson (1959).

Returning to encephalitides of known aetiology I will only say that our single British arbovirus, louping ill, causes very few human infections. But the closely related tick-borne encephalitis (TBE) virus, like louping ill a member of the B group of arboviruses, is widespread in continental Europe and has been shown to be endemic not far from us on parts of the Norwegian coast.

LABORATORY DIAGNOSIS OF ARBOVIRUS INFECTIONS

Virus isolation
Virus isolation is seldom achieved. Methods used by European workers are described in several contributions from the Institute

of Virology at Bratislava (Blaškovič 1967) about TBE in Czecho-slovakia. Isolations were made from ticks (*Ixodes ricinus*), from the blood of small mammals and from the CSF of one of 14 patients with meningoencephalitis. Injection of clarified material intracerebrally in suckling mice (aged 1 to 4 days) was more successful than isolation in chick embryo cell (CEC) culture. In the latter a cytopathic effect (CPE) was sometimes seen in two to three days. When no CPE was seen, TBE virus in the cultures could be made manifest by its prevention by interference of the CPE produced, in control cultures, by western equine encephalitis (WEE) virus used as challenge. Blind passages were made in both suckling mice and CEC cultures.

Isolates were identified by using them as antigens in haemag-glutination inhibition and complement fixation tests against known specific antisera. A method of identifying isolates in CEC cultures by an indirect fluorescent antibody method is described by 2 of the workers (Albrecht & Kŏzuch 1967). Type-specific antisera pre-pared in guinea-pigs against TBE and other group B arboviruses were applied to CEC cells either smeared on slides or growing on coverslips 5 days after they had been infected with the isolate. The preparations were then treated with a fluorescein-conjugated anti-guinea-pig globulin made in rabbits. Albrecht and Kŏzuch state that in positive preparations 'only a small proportion of the cells showed fluorescence' but this was sufficiently intense for identification. The same technique can be used with sections of infected mouse brain; the mice should be left till moribund before harvesting their brains.

Antibody in the serum of patients

The Czech workers used a test for *neutralizing antibody* to TBE virus described by Libiková (1963). Two-fold dilutions of patient's serum were left with a known constant dose of TBE virus for 18 hours at 4°C. A suspension of cynomologus monkey heart cells in Earle's saline with lactalbumin hydrolysate, inactivated horse serum and antibiotics was then added to the neutralization mix-tures, which were inspected for CPE or its inhibition after 5 days incubation at 37°C.

Haemagglutination inhibition (HI) tests by the method of Clarke and Casals (1958) are frequently used. Chick or goose erythrocytes are the most sensitive cells. Non-specific (lipid) inhibitors must be removed from sera by ether extraction before testing (Hirst 1965) and pH and temperature must be carefully controlled.

Complement fixation (CF) tests are sometimes more helpful than neutralization or HI tests in the diagnosis of current infection because CF antibody takes longer to develop and wanes more rapidly than HI or neutralizing antibody, so that a change in titre is more likely to be detected by the CF test. A method has been described by Casals et al. (1951).

A group in Minneapolis (Balfour et al. 1973) who diagnosed 66 cases of California encephalitis in 6 years by a change in HI or CF antibody titre, remark on the value of the gel-precipitin test (Wellings et al. 1970) in confirmation of recent infection with this virus when only one serum specimen is available. Precipitins become detectable about the fifth day of illness, reach a peak in one to three months and cannot be found after one year.

Standard methods for the laboratory investigation of arbovirus encephalitides are described in the American Public Health Association's *Diagnostic Procedures for Viral and Rickettsial Infections* (Hammon & Work 1964; Work 1964).

HERPES SIMPLEX ENCEPHALITIS

Clinical pathology

The peripheral blood   Unless the encephalitis is complicated by respiratory infection or intercurrent illness, there are no remarkable changes.

The cerebrospinal fluid   At first examination the CSF is normal in 12% of cases. In a further 12% leucocytes are fewer than 7/mm³ and protein less than 53 mg/100 ml. More usually 50–100 leucocytes, predominantly lymphocytes, are found. When serial examinations are made the cell count may increase during the first 2 to 3 weeks of illness: the protein often increases throughout the illness. Erythrocytes are found, even after atraumatic lumbar puncture, in 40% of cases, and xanthochromia in 11%. In aseptic meningitis, without cerebral involvement, shown by an increase in serum antibody to have been associated with herpes simplex virus, a lymphocytosis of about 300/mm³ and a protein of 60–70 mg/ 100 ml is usual (Illis & Gostling 1972). Low CSF chloride levels have been reported in herpes simplex encephalitis in 63% of 19 cases, whose mean chloride level was 111 mEq/litre, as against 104 mEq/litre in 10 cases of tuberculous meningitis and 123 mEq/litre in 19 adults with non-herpetic meningoencephalitis (Abramsky et al. 1971). The reduced chloride was not associated with low blood chloride. Low CSF glucose (< 45 mg/100 ml) was noted in 3 of the 19 cases of Abramsky et al. (1971) and in a case at the Massachusetts General Hospital (Castleman & McNeely 1971). One of the 6 cases of aseptic meningitis attributed to herpes simplex by Adair et al. (1953) had a CSF glucose of 10 mg/100 ml.

Diagnostic criteria

The proceedings of the Manchester symposium on acute necrotizing encephalitis were recently published (Longson 1973a). At that meeting it was agreed to set up a multi-centre trial of an antiviral chemotherapeutic substance in cases of herpes simplex encephalitis. The participants later agreed upon diagnostic criteria which must be satisfied by cases before they could be entered in the trial. These criteria include the isolation of herpes simplex virus from brain biopsy material or cerebrospinal fluid (usually ventricular) early in the patient's illness or the demonstration by microscopy of herpes virus or a herpes simplex virus antigen in brain biopsy material.

Virological procedures

The methods of virological diagnosis to be used in the trial have been agreed by the participants. As they represent the consensus of contemporary opinion about laboratory methods of making an aetiological diagnosis in cases of herpes simplex encephalitis they will be reproduced here.

1. *Specimens*
   a. *Brain biopsy*. To be collected in a dry sterile container. If the specimen is to be transferred to a distant laboratory, a small screw-capped bottle might help in minimising desiccation. Transport of the container to the distant laboratory should be in wet ice.
   b. *Ventricular fluid* in a dry sterile container. Transport of the container to a distant laboratory should be in wet ice.
   c. *Lumbar fluid* in a dry sterile container. Transport of the container to a distant laboratory should be in wet ice.
   d. *Throat swab, nasopharyngeal aspirate, faeces,* etc., at the discretion of the virologist.
   e. *Blood.* 10 ml clotted blood in a dry sterile container.
   Note: The transfer of all specimens for virus isolation and immunofluorescence should be as prompt as possible.

2. *Immunofluorescence*. Telephone contact with the laboratory concerned should be made as early as possible. Arrangements for transport and testing will be made between the persons concerned. The exact procedure for the immunofluorescent test is left to the discretion of the reference laboratory. The procedures which may be used are:

a. That described by Flewett (1973). The surface of the biopsy is pressed gently several times onto the surface of one or more microscope slides. When dry the preparations are fixed for 1 minute exactly in chilled (−20°C) acetone; longer fixation reduces the intensity of fluorescence.

All acetone must be allowed to evaporate before overlaying the slides with hyperimmune rabbit anti-herpes serum, for half an hour at 37°C in a wet chamber. After washing, appropriately diluted fluorescein-labelled anti-rabbit-globulin serum at PH 7·6 is applied for half an hour. The preparations are washed with buffered saline at pH 7·8 and mounted in glycerol buffered at pH 8·0. Flewett stresses that these recommended pH values are important for success: he also comments that the method avoids making frozen sections of unfixed brain and the attendant risk of cutting the fingers with a knife contaminated by encephalitogenic virus.

b. That described by Longson (1973b) which he points out is based on the method developed by Tomlinson (Tomlinson 1972; Tomlinson & MacCallum 1969). Biopsy material is mounted on the cryostat chuck, quenched with isopentane or liquid nitrogen and sectioned at 3–5 μm. On slides the sections are air dried and fixed for 10 minutes in anhydrous acetone. They may be stored at $-20°C$, sent through the mail to another laboratory or stained straight away. Longson (1973b) uses a fluorescein-conjugated anti-herpes rabbit serum for direct staining. The serum is obtained from a young, intensely immunized rabbit. The sera of many such rabbits may have to be conjugated and tested before a satisfactory one is obtained, for the antibody content of serum before con-jugation is no guide to its satisfactory performance after con-jugation. The method of conjugation follows that of Clark and Sheppard (1963). Longson emphasizes the great importance of achieving specificity, both by using the conjugated antiserum at a dilution which is high enough to involve some loss of brilliance in the specific fluorescence seen; and also by the inclusion of adequate controls. He also describes in detail the optical system which he favours.

3. *Virus isolation*
   a. *Brain biopsy.* Grind (e.g. in a Griffith's tube) in 2·0–2·5 ml of tissue culture medium (see below). Inoculate tissue cultures (see below) at the rate of 0·2 ml of suspension per tube. Centrifuge suspension in level centrifuge at 2000 rpm. Inoculate further tissue with supernatant at the rate of 0·2 ml per tube.

      Individual laboratories may wish to set up cultures of the actual brain tissue. The procedure for this is left to the discretion of the virologist.
   b. *Ventricular and lumbar fluids.* Inoculate tissue cultures (see below) at the rate of 0·1–0·2 ml per tube.
   c. *Other specimens.* At the discretion of the virologist.

4. *Tissue culture*
   a. *Cells.* The following cells are *recommended:*
      Human embryo fibroblasts
      Primary human amnion
      The following cell lines are NOT *recommended:*
      HeLa, H.Ep 2, KB
   b. *Medium.* No particular recommendation. The following medium has been found satisfactory for the maintenance of both human embryo fibroblasts and human amnion:

Eagle's medium B.M.E.	97·5%
Fetal calf serum	2·5%
Sodium bicarbonate	2·5 ml of 4·4%
Antibiotics	

   c. *Maintenance.* The tubes are maintained stationary. The cultures are washed and the medium changed 4 to 12 hours after inoculation, and thereafter at 3 to 4-day intervals. The cultures are examined for CPE twice daily for the first 72 hours, and thereafter daily.

5. *Identification of isolate* by routine neutralization procedure using specific antiserum. It might be found advisable to dilute the virus inoculum in order to obtain CPE in control cultures in a minimum of 3 days. The anti-serum is used at a dilution which is found to retard significantly the onset of CPE in the test culture.

In cases of doubt, it will be necessary to prepare a suspension of virus containing 100 TCD 50/0.1 ml, of isolate and to test this against 0·1 ml of progressive dilutions of antiserum.

6. *Serology* by standard CFT procedures.

Dayan and Stokes (1973) have suggested that the need to enter the skull can be eliminated by fluorescence microscopy of deposited leucocytes of lumbar cerebrospinal fluid. Dayan has reported the identification of virus antigen in such cells in cases of herpes simplex and SSPE. He and his colleague also describe the recognition of cells producing immunoglobulins and imply that the presence of such cells is indicative of infection of the brain substance. These claims, though partially supported by Gupta (1973), have been criticized (Longson et al. 1973) on the grounds that a firm aetiological diagnosis must be made before exhibiting cytotoxic drugs in suspected cases of herpes simplex encephalitis.

Reading the reported discussion of the Manchester symposium one finds that not all participants were persuaded that cytotoxic drugs should wait upon firm diagnosis. Professor Hall (1973), an oncologist, of Rochester, N.Y., said these drugs were feared unreasonably. He advocated treatment on suspicion of herpes simplex encephalitis while waiting for laboratory confirmation and he was supported by Ross (1973) of the Glasgow Regional Virus Laboratory. Many physicians confronted with a suspected case are so situated that they must initiate treatment before confirmation of the diagnosis or deny their patient the admittedly debatable benefits of antiviral therapy for several days.

CASE REPORT

The most recent case of herpes simplex encephalitis confirmed in our laboratory was treated on the basis of a clinical diagnosis.

25 February 1974. A 57-year-old lorry driver living in West Sussex who had been treated with acetazolamide (Diamox) for glaucoma for some years, but who had never had cold sores, complained of dizziness at lunch. He retired to bed and his wife noticed that he was grinding his teeth and foaming at the mouth. His doctor found his temperature was 37·8°C (100°F) and prescribed paracetemol. He slept.

26 February 1974. He was conscious and aware of his surroundings. His doctor found him confused and complaining of headache. His temperature was 37·9°C (100·2°F) and blood pressure 140/80. When protruded his tongue wobbled. There were no other abnormal physical signs.

27 February 1974. He was anorexic and behaved strangely. His doctor found cerebral irritation and suspected ENCEPHALITIS. He was admitted to hospital. The admitting doctor found him confused and red-eyed and also diagnosed ENCEPHALITIS. Blood leucocytes were 12 000/mm³, with neutrophils 92%. Cerebrospinal fluid showed 40 lymphocytes, and protein 65 mg. The EEG was recorded. Treatment was sedation.

28 February 1974. He was dysarthric. His pulse rate, temperature and blood pressure were rising. Cerebrospinal fluid: Cells, 56 lymphocytes; protein 75 mg; glucose 80 mg. A neurosurgeon was consulted by telephone and the following treatment was administered: dexamethasone 5 mg 6-hourly; cytosine arabinoside 50 mg intrathecally and cytosine arabinoside 100 mg 12-hourly intravenously; Idoxuridine 3·25 g in 2 litres of fluid intravenously.

4 March 1974. By this day he had had a further 12 g of idoxuridine in 8 litres of fluid and this drug was stopped.

5 March 1974. His temperature was normal and he seemed better though not oriented. His right pupil was larger than his left. Plantar responses were flexor. Dexamethasone dose reduced to 5 mg 8-hourly.

7 March 1974. He was worse and could not recognize his wife. Cerebrospinal fluid: cells, 40 lymphocytes; protein, 120 mg. Cytosine arabinoside 50 mg intrathecally was given.

10 March 1974. He had epileptiform seizures starting on the right side.

11 March 1974. Cerebrospinal fluid: pressure, 230 mmHg; cells, 17 lymphocytes; protein, 120 mg.

13 March 1974. Intravenous cytosine arabinoside stopped. His condition continued to deteriorate and he had stridor and râles at both bases.

15 March 1974. He died.

Herpesvirus hominis was isolated from a piece of temporal lobe of his brain, taken at post-mortem examination.

It is interesting that specific treatment was begun within 3 days of the onset of illness, with both idoxuridine and cytarabine as well as dexamethasone. However, treatment not only failed to prevent a fatal outcome, but did not prevent recovery of live virus from the brain after death on the nineteenth day of illness.

Table 9 shows the results of tests for antibody on specimens of serum and cerebrospinal fluid. The patient had some serum antibody on the seventh day of illness and it did not increase significantly during the next 11 days.

TABLE 9

TITRE OF ANTIBODY TO *Herpesvirus hominis* IN A PATIENT
WITH HERPES SIMPLEX ENCEPHALITIS

| Date | Serum | | | Cerebrospinal fluid | | |
| | Neutralization | | Comple-ment fixation | Neutralization | | Comple-ment fixation |
	Type 1	Type 2		Type 1	Type 2	
28 Feb. 1974	—	—	—	<4	<4	2
3 March 1974	64	>4	32	—	—	—
7 March 1974	128	4	64	<4	<4	2
11 March 1974	—	—	—	<4	<4	8
14 March 1974	128	4	64	—	—	—

Onset 25 Feb. 1974; death 15 March 1974.

There is still argument as to whether or not herpes simplex encephalitis is nearly always a primary infection: in this patient's case the serological evidence could support Longson's contention (personal communication) that this disease is usually a recurrence. Alternatively the treatment, begun so commendably early and some of it continued till the end, may have interfered with antibody production, preventing the achievement of the very high peak titre so often seen. Although antibody may not appear or increase until after the twelfth day of this disease (and indeed there are reports (Lerner et al. 1971) of the titre rising for the first time nearly 30 days after the onset of illness), it has then increased rapidly; this patient's titre was still unchanged on the eighteenth day of disease.

Kurtz (1974), who has examined the sera and cerebrospinal fluids of patients with herpes simplex encephalitis for IgG and IgM antibody against herpes simplex virus, has found serum IgM antibody responses like those in primary non-encephalitic herpes simplex in 8 of 9 adult patients, but no IgM antibody in their CSF.

In this patient there was no early appearance of antibody in the cerebrospinal fluid. But the last specimen was collected only 15 days after the onset of illness: titres of complement fixing antibody in the CSF greater than 16 have not been recorded before the twelfth day of illness (MacCallum et al. 1974).

Laboratory diagnosis of viral encephalitis

Unfortunately it is not possible to extol the helpfulness of the laboratory in the diagnosis of viral encephalitis. But, excepting the diagnosis of herpes simplex by examination of brain biopsy, the laboratory diagnosis of encephalitis is likely to be made some weeks after the onset of the illness.

I am grateful to Dr Hinton, the physician in charge of the patient, for permission to report this case, and to Dr Michael Nicholls, of the microbiology laboratory which received the specimen in the first place, for extracting from the notes the chronological record of the patient's illness.

REFERENCES

Abramsky, O., Carmon, A. & Feldman, S. (1971) Cerebrospinal fluid in acute necrotizing encephalitis: hypochlorrhachia as a diagnostic aid. *J. neurol. Sci.*, **14**, 183.

Acheson, E. D. (1959) The clinical syndrome variously called benign myalgic encephalomyelitis, Iceland disease and epidemic neuromyasthenia. *Am. J. Med.*, **26**, 569.

Adair, C. V., Gauld, R. L. & Smadel, J. E. (1953) Aseptic meningitis, a disease of diverse etiology: clinical and etiologic studies on 854 cases. *Am. J. intern. Med.*, **39**, 675.

Albrecht, P. & Kŏzuch, O. (1967) Rapid identification of tick-borne encephalitis virus by the fluorescent antibody technique. *Bull. Wld Hlth Org.*, **36**, Suppl. 1, 85.

Balfour, H. H., jun., Siem, R. A., Bauer, H. & Quie, P. G. (1973) California arbovirus (La Crosse) infections: I. Clinical and laboratory findings in 66 children with meningoencephalitis. *Pediatrics, Springfield*, **52**, 680.

Blaškovič, D. (1967) Studies on tick-borne encephalitis. *Bull. Wld Hlth Org.*, **36**, Suppl. 1.

Bower, B. D. (1969) The problem of acute encephalopathy in children. In *Virus Diseases and the Nervous System*, ed. Whitty, C. W. M., Hughes, J. T. & MacCallum, F. O., p. 48. Oxford: Blackwell Scientific.

Casals, J., Olitsky, P. K. & Anslow, R. O. (1951) A specific complement fixation test for infection with poliomyelitis virus. *J. exp. Med.*, **94**, 123.

Castleman, B. & McNeely, B. U. (1971) Case records of the Massachusetts general hospital: weekly clinicopathological exercises. *New Engl. J. Med.*, **281**, 1023.

Clark, H. F. & Sheppard, C. C. (1963) A dialysis technique for preparing fluorescent antibody. *Virology*, **20**, 642.

Clarke, D. H. & Casals, J. (1958) Techniques for hemagglutination and hemagglutination-inhibition with arthropod-borne viruses. *Am. J. trop. Med. Hyg.*, **7**, 561.

Dayan, A. D. & Stokes, M. I. (1973) Rapid diagnosis of encephalitis by immunofluorescent examination of cerebrospinal fluid cells. *Lancet*, **i**, 177.

Findlay, L. & Shiskin, C. (1921) Epidemic encephalitis (encephalitis lethargica) in childhood: with special reference to the changes in the cerebrospinal fluid. *Glasg. med. J.*, 3.

Flewett, T. H. (1973) The rapid diagnosis of herpes encephalitis. *Postgrad. med. J.*, **49**, 398.

Galpine, J. F. & Brady, C. (1957) Benign myalgic encephalomyelitis. *Lancet*, **i**, 757.

Gupta, P. K. (1973) Cytodiagnosis of viral encephalitis. *Lancet*, **i**, 609.

Hall, T. C. (1973) Therapy of herpes simplex encephalitis. *Postgrad. med. J.*, **49**, 438.

Hammon, W. McD. & Work, T. H. (1964) Arbovirus infection in man. In *Diagnostic Procedures for Viral and Rickettsial Diseases*, ed. Lennette, E. H. & Schmidt, N. J., 3rd ed., p. 268. New York: American Public Health Association.

Helle, I. (1972) Newer diagnostic and therapeutic methods in meningitis and encephalitis. *Acta neurol. scand.*, **48**, Suppl. 51, 305.

Henle, W. & Enders, J. F. (1965) Mumps virus. In *Viral and Rickettsial Infections of Man*, ed. Horsfall, F. L. & Tamm, I., p. 760. Philadelphia: Lippincott.

Hirst, G. K. (1965) Cell-virus attachment and the action of antibodies on viruses. In *Viral and Rickettsial Infections of Man*, ed. Horsfall, F. L. & Tamm, I., p. 220. Philadelphia: Lippincott.

Illis, L. S. & Gostling, J. V. T. (1972) *Herpes Simplex Encephalitis*, p. 40. Bristol: Scientechnica.

Innes, S. G. B. (1970) Encephalomyelitis resembling benign myalgic encephalomyelitis. *Lancet*, **i**, 969.

Kennedy, C. & Wanglee, P. (1967) Encephalitis: a variable syndrome in response to viral infection. *Pediat. Clins N. Am.*, **14**, 809.

Kurtz, J. B. (1974) Specific IgG and IgM antibody responses in herpes simplex virus infections. *J. med. Microbiol.*, **7**, 333.

Lerner, A. M., Bailey, E. J. & Nolan, D. C. (1970) Complement-requiring neutralizing antibodies in *Herpesvirus hominis* encephalitis. *J. Immunol.*, **104**, 607.

Libíková, H. (1963) Assay of the tick-borne encephalitis virus in HeLa cells. III. Selection and properties of virus antigens for an *in vitro* neutralization test. *Acta virol.*, **7**, 516.

Longson, M. (1937a) Acute necrotizing encephalitis and other herpes simplex virus infections. *Postgrad. med. J.*, **49**, 371.

Longson, M. (1973b) Immunofluorescence in the diagnosis of herpes encephalitis. *Postgrad. med. J.*, **49**, 403.

Longson, M., Liversedge, L. A. & Wilkinson, I. M. S. (1973) Diagnosis of virus encephalitis. *Lancet*, **i**, 371.

MacCallum, F. O., Chinn, I. J. & Gostling, J. V. T. (1974) Antibodies to herpes simplex virus in the cerebrospinal fluid of patients with herpetic encephalitis. *J. med. Microbiol.*, **7**, 325,

McEvedy, C. P. & Beard, A. W. (1970). Concept of benign myalgic encephalomyelitis. *Br. med. J.*, **i**, 11.

McKendrick, G. D. W. (1968) Encephalitis. *Lancet*, **i**, 1248.

Miller, J. R. & Harter, D. H. (1972) Acute viral encephalitis. *Med. Clins N. Am.*, **56**, 1393.

Ramsay, A. M. (1957) Encephalomyelitis in north west London: An endemic infection simulating poliomyelitis and hysteria. *Lancet*, **ii**, 1196.

Richardson, A. T. (1956) Some aspects of the Royal Free Hospital epidemic. *Ann. phys. Med.*, **3**, 81.

Ross, C. A. C. (1973) Therapy of herpes simplex encephalitis. *Postgrad. med. J.*, **49**, 438.

Scott, T. F. McN. (1969) Encephalitis. In *Text Book of Pediatrics*, ed. Nelson, W. E., Vaughan, V. C. & McKay, R. J., 9th ed., p. 690. Philadelphia: Saunders.

Tomlinson, A. H. (1972) Tungsten halogen lamps and interference filters for immunofluorescent microscopy. *Proc. R. microsc. Soc.*, **7**, 1.

Tomlinson, A. H. & MacCallum, F. O. (1969) Virological diagnosis of herpes simplex encephalitis. In *Virus Diseases and the Nervous System*, ed. Whitty, C. W. M., Hughes, J. T. & MacCallum, F. O., p. 21. Oxford: Blackwell Scientific.

Wellings, F. M., Sather, G. C. & Hammon, W. McD. (1970) A type-specific immunodiffusion technique for the California encephalitis virus group. *J. Immunol.*, **105**, 1194.

Work, T. H. (1964) Isolation and identification of arthropod-borne viruses. In *Diagnostic Procedures for Viral and Rickettsial Diseases*, ed. Lennette, E. H. & Schmidt, N. J., p. 312. New York: American Public Health Association.

5

Electroencephalographic Changes in Viral Encephalitis

W. A. COBB

Information regarding the EEG of acute viral encephalitides is relatively scanty and the majority of papers are concerned with small groups or single cases. Nevertheless a fairly consistent pattern emerges.

Measles
In the encephalitis complicating infection with the non-neurotropic viruses the EEG is usually severely abnormal, perhaps in part because the majority of the patients are young. The most studied has been measles, in which there is usually loss of all normal activity and its replacement by widespread slow waves; their absence was thought by Levy and Roseman (1954) to make the diagnosis most unlikely. Radermecker (1956) pointed out a relationship between the amount of slow activity and the state of drowsiness. Return of the EEG to normality is usually very slow.

It is of interest that Pampiglione (1964), recording during the acute stage of uncomplicated measles, found changes which could not be attributed to fever or intoxication, suggesting the possibility of clinically unsuspected cerebral involvement.

Primary acute viral encephalitis

The different forms of primary acute viral encephalitis do not appear to give rise to individually characteristic EEG changes and the commonest picture is one of diffuse slow activity, though focal changes are not infrequent. Hanzal (1959) reports on 42 patients with 'tick encephalitis', of whom 10 had focal EEG changes. On the other hand, there were 12 with normal EEGs but it appears that a significant proportion of these 42 patients did not have encephalitic signs at the time of the EEG. Grabow et al. (1969) describe the EEG in 45 cases of 'California arbovirus' encephalitis but only 13 of the patients were seen in the first month of illness; these all had generalized slow activity, some with focal features as well.

Herpes simplex encephalitis

These unspecific findings are in great contrast with the EEG of herpes simplex encephalitis, first described by Radermecker in 1956; at the same time he reported similar findings in cases of acute necrotizing encephalitis which, as he suspected, has proved to be the same disease. The probable specificity of the EEG was first recognized by Millar and Coey (1959); further cases have been reported by Drachman and Adams (1962), Rawls et al. (1966) and Adams and Jennett (1967) among others.

The characteristic features of the EEG of herpes simplex encephalitis were stressed particularly by Vincent et al. (1969) and Upton and Gumpert (1970) and have proved to be of great early diagnostic value, though some authors have denied their importance (Illis & Taylor 1972). They are the rapid disruption and slowing of background activity with the appearance, on the second to about the fifteenth day of illness, of repetitive, nearly stereotyped, slow wave discharges from one or other temporal region (Fig. 2). Each discharge is usually a single and rather simple slow wave with a duration up to 1 second and they repeat with fairly constant form and interval, usually 1–4 seconds. As the disease progresses the repetitive feature may become less clear and the amplitude of the background slow activity may diminish;

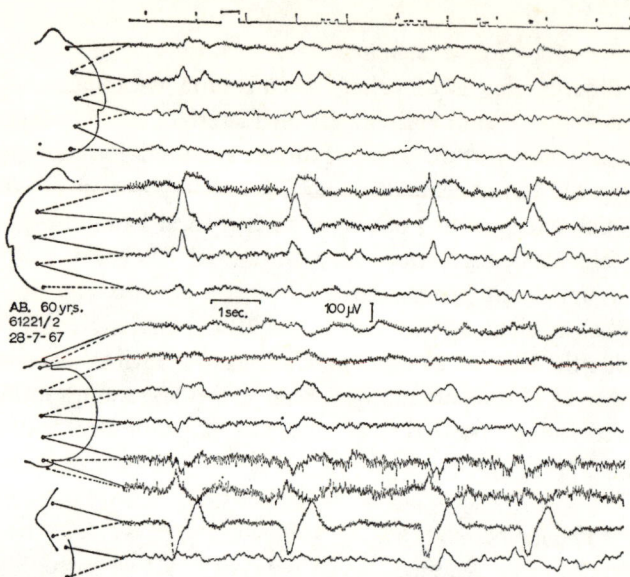

Fig. 2. Herpes simplex encephalitis in a 60-year-old man on the ninth day of illness.

Radermecker (1956) suggested that the EEG might become more normal on the first affected side but it seems more likely that it becomes relatively inactive as necrosis proceeds. Meanwhile the electrical activity of the second temporal region may go through the same series of events, if death does not intervene, and sometimes the two hemispheres may be seen to produce similar, independent, repetitive discharges.

Discharges of this kind were seen in about half the reported cases, often with a single EEG, and the proportion is certainly much higher when they are looked for daily from the onset of disease. In one of our cases in which they did not appear the disease had an unusual distribution, being largely confined to the brain stem. Thus, although the picture is not invariably found, it is extremely frequent and of high diagnostic value in an acute cerebral illness.

Gupta and Seth (1973) have reported that when herpes simplex virus of either type I or II is injected into the brains of rabbits an acute lethal encephalitis develops which is accompanied, from the fifth day, by periodic discharges with a usual interval of 2–2·5 seconds.

Regular periodic events have not been noted in any other type of acute human encephalitis but they do occur in at least two types of viral infection in laboratory animals. Regular massive myoclonic jerks were found by Luttrel and Bang (1956) in cats infected with Newcastle disease virus, and these continued after section of the spinal cord, showing that cerebral connections were not necessary for their maintenance. Further, when pseudo-rabies virus is injected into the eye of the rat, infection of the superior cervical ganglion results; it gives rise to bursts of action potentials at a fairly regular interval of 2–3 seconds (Dempsher et al. 1955). These continue after removal of the ganglion, indicating that no complex circuitry is necessary to bring the cells into approximate synchrony and to maintain their regular firing at relatively long intervals, observations which may be of the greatest importance to the understanding of the mechanisms involved in regular discharges.

Subacute sclerosing panencephalitis
Such discharges had in fact been noted some years earlier in clinical cases, in the subacute sclerosing leucoencephalitis of van Bogaert by Radermecker (1949) and in the inclusion body encephalitis of Dawson by Cobb and Hill (1950). Though uncommon, this has proved to be the most characteristic and specific of EEG phenomena and there is a quite large literature concerned with it, from which Hamoen et al. (1956), Radermecker and Poser (1960), Storm van Leeuwen (1964) and Cobb (1966) might be mentioned. At the time when the EEG was first described it was by no means certain that the two diseases were manifestations of the same illness and their viral nature was only suggested by the intranuclear inclusion bodies found in the Dawson form.

The feature which characterizes the EEG of subacute sclerosing panencephalitis (SSPE) is a nearly stereotyped complex, predominantly of slow waves, which recurs at nearly regular intervals throughout long periods of the disease (Fig. 3). The complex

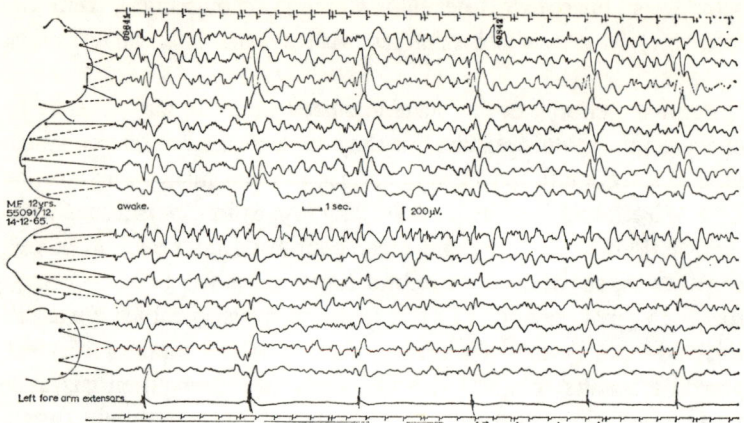

Fig. 3. A 12-year-old boy in the seventh month of SSPE, from which he died 8 months later. The waking EEG, showing a generalized stereotyped complex repeating at 5½-second intervals on a grossly abnormal background. Each complex is accompanied by a very brief EMG discharge from the left forearm extensors.

varies greatly from subject to subject, in some being relatively brief (0·5 second) and simple and in others more or less prolonged (2·5 seconds) and complicated; not only does its form vary with the subject but also from day to day and with the state of wakefulness. It must therefore be stressed that its characteristic is the similarity between complexes in a given case at any one time. Occasionally complexes occur at rare and irregular intervals but they usually soon settle at an interval of about 8 seconds, with a range from case to case and time to time of 3 to about 20 seconds; intervals of less than 4 and more than 12 seconds are in fact rare. In a given case the mean interval may change from day to day or be rather constant; on any occasion there are usually a few intervals which are notably long or short but the majority will be within 20% of the mean. Both the form and the interval may be different in sleep, changing rapidly on waking.

Complexes may commence very early in the illness (Cobb 1966) though they are more usually delayed for a few months; their onset is often simultaneous with the appearance of rhythmic jerking. They may at first be predominant on one or other side, usually without any clear clinical asymmetry, and thereafter become widespread and roughly synchronous on the two sides, even though the wave form is usually very different from one area to another. Once established, the complexes tend to continue until death, sometimes throughout long remissions; not infrequently, however, they disappear for a time, only to be seen again at the next examination. A possible explanation of this erratic behaviour is to be found in the observation by Farrell et al. (1971) that complexes could be abolished by an induced rise in body temperature, by as little as 0·5°C in one case; cooling resulted in an increased frequency of the complexes. Exceptionally, complexes can be evoked by stimuli and this seems to occur when their presence is inconstant, either at their first appearance or when returning after an absence.

The background on which these complexes appear shows progressive changes, with loss of alpha rhythm and increasing slow activity, usually widespread but sometimes showing a local maximum which may be in agreement with the clinical signs. Sometimes the delta waves remit momentarily after each complex; otherwise the two main components of the EEG appear to be independent. Similarly, in the few reports of recorded epileptic attacks, the complexes appear to be unrelated to the epileptic discharge. In occasional cases (Cobb 1966) there has been very little change in background activity to within a few days of death.

Motor disturbances are the rule in SSPE and among these there is nearly always one which is time-locked to the complex; it is usually a stereotyped myoclonic jerk, which may involve much of the body, though it can be limited to a single digit. Less commonly the recurrent disturbance is inhibitory, involving voluntary or spontaneous activity, including posture. Thus the electromyogram of appropriate muscles provides important confirmation of the EEG evidence for SSPE. However, complexes can occur without jerks; they frequently do so early in the disease and always during sleep. The converse, jerks without complexes, also occurs, though rarely (Petsche et al. 1961).

Many unsuccessful attempts were made to cultivate a virus or infect a laboratory animal with material from SSPE brains, even before it became apparent that measles or a closely related virus was the responsible agent (Connolly et al. 1967; Legg 1967; Baublis & Payne 1968; Sever & Zeman 1968; Horta-Barbosa et al. 1969). Recently, however, Notermans et al. (1973) have been able to infect beagle puppies by intracerebral injection of brain cell culture from a case of human SSPE (though not of wild measles virus). The puppies not only developed a disease showing 'a close resemblance to the human disease' but their EEGs contained periodic complexes.

Jakob–Creutzfeldt disease

A second subacute disease in which repetitive EEG discharges are almost invariably found was first described by Jones and Nevin (1954) as subacute vascular encephalopathy and by Pallis and Spillane (1957) as subacute progressive encephalopathy, now generally assimilated under the title of Jakob–Creutzfeldt disease. Gibbs et al. (1968) were able to produce a very similar disease, with a long latency, by inoculating affected human brain material into the brains of chimpanzees and, later, from them to New World monkeys (Gajdusek & Gibbs 1971).

The human disease runs a course of 3–12 months, with steadily progressive dementia leading to coma and with involuntary movements, often including repetitive myoclonus. The EEG is disturbed early, with loss of normal activity and the presence of generalized slow waves. The specific picture (Fig. 4) has usually developed by the time there is severe disturbance of consciousness; it consists in the nearly regular recurrence, at an interval which is commonly rather less than 1 second, of a relatively simple sharp wave lasting up to 0·5 second. It is not completely stereotyped, often having several forms in the given case, ranging from nearly monophasic, through the commonest triphasic form, to occasionally more polyphasic ones. When regular jerks are present they are associated with these sharp waves in time. Late in the disease the sharp waves may be replaced by moderate voltage slow activity, but can be restored by arousing stimuli. Sometimes

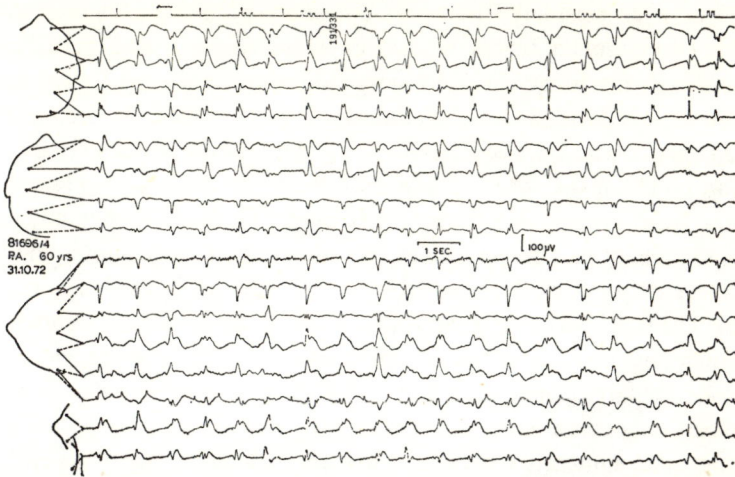

Fig. 4. Jakob–Creutzfeldt disease. A 60-year-old woman in the third month of increasing dementia, leading to coma.

the sharp waves are initially quite local though they always later become widespread.

Some two years before their report on the transmission of Jakob–Creutzfeldt disease to chimpanzees Gajdusek et al. (1966, 1967) had reported a similar success in kuru, the pathology of which can also be described as that of a subacute spongiform encephalopathy. For this reason we recorded the EEG of the majority of living patients with kuru (Cobb et al. 1973); that they were only mildly abnormal (and never periodic) even in the late stages may perhaps be attributed to the fact that the maximal incidence is on the cerebellum, which is poorly represented in the EEG.

PERIODIC COMPLEXES

Attempts to find an anatomical basis for the periodicity of SSPE have been unsuccessful (Guazzi 1961; Osetowska 1961) and are still less likely to succeed if a common explanation is sought to cover the three human diseases in which periodicity is the rule.

When it is considered that periodic cerebral discharge is seen in the experimental forms of two of these diseases and periodic neuronal discharge in laboratory infections with two further viruses it is difficult to escape the conclusion that viral or viral-like infection is the common factor. With the pseudo-rabies preparation of Dempsher et al. (1955) as a model it could be supposed that large groups of infected cells might be made to fire autorhythmically and in approximate synchrony. The resultant discharge might itself be recordable in the EEG (in herpes simplex, for example) or might activate, directly or indirectly, cortex which might or might not be still unaffected. The latter projected mode is particularly probable in SSPE in which periodic complexes may commence very early in the disease and persist for a long time, sometimes with little evidence of cortical involvement. The near constancy of the discharges on any occasion allows of very little variation at that time in the trigger zone, the paths of spread from it and the sequence of activation of the cortex.

SSPE, Jakob–Creutzfeldt disease and herpes simplex encephalitis are the only three human diseases in which periodic complexes can be expected to occur. Nevertheless such complexes are seen as rare and unpredictable accompaniments of a number of other cerebral conditions, of which the following are least uncommon. Occasional hemisphere lesions of all kinds, but particularly tumours and infarcts, give rise to focal repetitive discharges, usually with an interval of 1–4 seconds; commonly they are seen only for a few days during an acute phase of what may be a prolonged illness. They were first described by Lecasble and Dondey (1957) and in greater detail by Chatrian et al. (1964), who found a strong, if not complete, association with epilepsy, though not with the actual occurrence of attacks, apart from epilepsia partialis continua in a few cases. There is nothing obvious which distinguishes these cases from the far more numerous tumours and infarcts which are not associated with periodic discharges. Chatrian et al., in 33 patients, found that 12 had severe fever, 12 were chronic alcoholics and 18 'had uraemia and/or disorders of fluid, electrolyte and acid-base balance', which suggests that a secondary factor in producing periodic discharges may be a disturbance of metabolism; personal experience however is that such disturbances need not be present.

Nevertheless one type of metabolic encephalopathy is often associated with triphasic waves: in hepatic coma (Bickford & Butt 1955) they are usually random but may recur regularly to form a picture not unlike that of Jakob–Creutzfeldt disease, particularly in its early stages before the pattern is fully developed. Based on the abolition of triphasic sharp waves by amantadine in one case of Jakob–Creutzfeldt disease and in one of acute hemiplegia due to infarction, Hamoen (1973) has suggested that these repetitive waves are 'caused by a disturbance of the dopaminergic function'.

A third situation in which repetitive discharges are sometimes transiently seen is during the recovery phase after an epileptic attack. After a major convulsion it is usual for the EEG to be of low voltage and for episodes of slow wave to occur on this flat background, gradually increasing in number until slow activity is continuous; usually these episodes are quite variable in content but occasionally they have a stereotyped and relatively simple form.

These three types of repetitive discharge and the still rarer ones with other diseases (see Gaches 1971) seldom cause any diagnostic problem. The most likely confusions are between the early asymmetric distribution in SSPE and the periodic discharge of a local lesion and between early Jakob–Creutzfeldt disease and hepatic coma. In the clinical context there is seldom difficulty in making the correct choice and the EEG has in fact a very high diagnostic value in these cases.

It is remarkable that the periodic complexes of SSPE, Jakob–Creutzfeldt disease and herpes simplex are quite distinctive, with little of overlap even in atypical cases, each having a range of wave forms and a rather narrow range of intervals which, in combination, distinguish it from the others. Since the destructive course of the disease does not change these ranges by much it seems unlikely that they have a simple anatomical basis (the interval between discharges, for example, might be determined by the path length of a retroactive circuit) and more probable that the periodicity represents the time constant of recovery of an electro-chemical process at the cell membrane, disturbed by the specific effect of 'virus' or of altered local metabolism. This relative autorhythmicity need not, of course, imply that the affected system would be entirely isolated from external influences, for example the triggering of complexes by stimuli in SSPE or their suppression by hyperthermia in the same disease. Gloor et al. (1968) express much the same idea in relation to a case of Heidenhain's disease with an EEG picture of the Jakob–Creutzfeldt type, in which the sharp waves could be triggered by auditory or visual stimuli at sufficiently long intervals, the response to a second flash being already much reduced at an interval of 600 mseconds.

Nevertheless, a degree of anatomical constancy does seem to be implicit in the relative lack of variation of the complexes, particularly in SSPE, because a given distribution and form of the waves must depend on the size, shape, orientation and sequence of activation of the ultimate cortical generators whose activity results in the recorded EEG.

REFERENCES

Adams, J. H. & Jennett, W. B. (1967) Acute necrotizing encephalitis: a problem of diagnosis. *J. Neurol. Neurosurg. Psychiat.*, **30**, 248.

Baublis, J. V. & Payne, F. E. (1968) Measles antigen and syncytium formation in brain cell cultures from subacute sclerosing panencephalitis (SSPE). *Proc. Soc. exp. Biol. N.Y.*, **129**, 593.

Bickford, R. G. & Butt, H. R. (1955) Hepatic coma: the electroencephalographic pattern. *J. clin. Invest.*, **34**, 790.

Chatrian, G. E., Shaw, C.-M. & Leffman, H. (1964) The significance of periodic lateralized epileptiform discharges in EEG: an electrographic, clinical and pathological study. *Electroenceph. clin. Neurophysiol.*, **17**, 177.

Cobb, W. A. (1966) The periodic events of subacute sclerosing leucoencephalitis. *Electroenceph. clin. Neurophysiol.*, **21**, 278.

Cobb, W. A. (1968) Depth recording in subacute sclerosing leucoencephalitis. In *Clinical Electroencephalography of Children*, ed. Kellaway, P. & Petersén, I. Stockholm: Almqvist & Wiksell.

Cobb, W. A. & Hill, D. (1950) Electroencephalogram in subacute progressive encephalitis. *Brain*, **73**, 392.

Cobb, W. A., Hornabrook, R. W. & Sanders, S. (1973) The EEG of kuru. *Electroenceph. clin. Neurophysiol.*, **34**, 419.

Connolly, J. H., Allen, I. V., Hurwitz, L. J. & Millar, J. H. D. (1967) Measles virus antibody and antigen in subacute sclerosing panencephalitis. *Lancet*, **i**, 542.

Dempsher, J., Larrabee, M. G., Bang, F. B. & Bodian, D. (1955) Physiological changes in sympathetic ganglia infected with pseudorabies virus. *Am. J. Physiol.*, **182**, 203.

Drachman, D. A. & Adams, R. D. (1962) Herpes simplex and acute inclusion-body encephalitis. *Archs Neurol., Chicago*, **7**, 45.

Farrell, D. F., Starr, A. & Freeman, J. M. (1971) The effect of body temperature on the 'periodic complexes' of subacute sclerosing leucoencephalitis (SSLE). *Electroenceph. clin. Neurophysiol.*, **30**, 415.

Gaches, J. (1971) Activités périodiques en EEG. *Rev. EEG neurophysiol.*, **1**, 9.

Gajdusek, D. C. & Gibbs, C. J., jun. (1971) Transmission of two subacute spongiform encephalopathies of man (kuru and Creutzfeld–Jakob disease) to New World monkeys. *Nature, Lond.*, **230**, 588.

Gajdusek, D. C., Gibbs, C. J., jun. & Alpers, M. (1966) Experimental transmission of a kuru-like syndrome to chimpanzees. *Nature, Lond.*, **209**, 794.

Gajdusek, D. C., Gibbs, C. J., jun. & Alpers, M. (1967) Transmission and passage of experimental 'kuru' to chimpanzees. *Science, N.Y.* **155**, 212.

Gibbs, C. J., jun., Gajdusek, D. C., Asher, D. M., Alpers, M. P., Beck, E., Daniel, P. M. & Matthews, W. B. (1968) Creutzfeld–Jakob disease (spongiform encephalopathy): transmission to the chimpanzee. *Science, N.Y.*, **161**, 388.

Gloor, P., Kalebay, O. & Giard, N. (1968) The electroencephalogram in diffuse encephalopathies: electroencephalographic correlates of grey and white matter lesions. *Brain*, **91**, 799.

Grabow, J. D., Matthews, C. G., Chun, R. W. & Thompson, W. H. (1969) The electroencephalogram and clinical sequelae of California arbovirus encephalitis. *Neurol., Minneap.*, **19**, 394.

Guazzi, G. C. (1961) The distribution of brainstem and medullary lesions in subacute sclerosing leucoencephalitis (pathological analysis of 50 cases). In *Encephalitides*, ed. van Bogaert, L., Radermecker, J., Hozay, J. & Lowenthal, A., pp. 471–92. Amsterdam: Elsevier.

Gupta, P. C. & Seth, P. (1973) Periodic complexes in herpes simplex encephalitis. A clinical and experimental study. *Electroenceph. clin. Neurophysiol.*, **35**, 67.

Hamoen, A.-M. (1973) Possible association between triphasic EEG waves and disorder of dopaminergic function. *Br. med. J.*, **ii**, 272.

Hamoen, A.-M., Herngreen, H., Storm van Leeuwen, W. & Magnus, O. (1956) Encéphalite subaiguë progressive, constatations cliniques et électroencéphalographiques dans 23 cas. *Rev. neurol.*, **94**, 109.

Hanzal, F. (1961) Biochemical and electroencephalographical aspects of tick encephalitis. In *Encephalitides*, ed. van Bogaert, L., Radermecker, J. Hozay, J. & Lowenthal, A., pp. 661–70. Amsterdam: Elsevier.

Horta-Barbosa, L., Fucillo, D. A., Sever, J. L. & Zeman, W. (1969)

Subacute sclerosing panencephalitis: isolation of measles virus from a brain biopsy. *Nature, Lond.*, **221**, 974.

Illis, L. S. & Taylor, F. M. (1972) The electroencephalogram in herpes simplex encephalitis. *Lancet*, **i**, 718.

Jones, D. P. & Nevin, S. (1954) Rapidly progressive cerebral degeneration (subacute vascular encephalopathy) with mental disorder, focal disturbances and myoclonic epilepsy. *J. Neurol. Neurosurg. Psychiat.*, **17**, 148.

Lecasble, R. & Dondey, M. (1957) Ondes lentes focalisées en succession pseudo-périodiques observées dans certaines néoformations cérébrales en évolution aiguë ou subaiguë. *Excerpta med.*, **37**, 120.

Legg, N. J. (1967) Virus antibodies in subacute sclerosing panencephalitis: a study of 22 patients. *Br. med. J.*, **iii**, 350.

Levy, L. L. & Roseman, E. (1954) Electroencephalographic studies of the encephalopathics. III. Measles. *Am. J. Dis. Childh.*, **88**, 5.

Luttrell, C. N. & Bang, F. B. (1956) Myoclonus in cats with Newcastle disease virus encephalitis. *Trans. Am. neurol. Ass.*, **81**, 59.

Millar, J. H. D. & Coey, A. (1959) The EEG in necrotizing encephalitis. *Electroenceph. clin. Neurophysiol.*, **11**, 582.

Notermans, S. L. H., Tijl, W. F. J., Willems, F. T. C. & Sloof, J. L. (1973) Experimentally induced subacute sclerosing panencephalitis in young dogs. *Neurology, Minneap.*, **23**, 543.

Osetowska, E. (1961) The distribution of telencephalic lesions in subacute sclerosing leucoencephalitis (pathological examination of 50 cases). In *Encephalitides*, ed. van Bogaert, L., Radermecker, J., Hozay, J. & Lowenthal, A., pp. 414–69. Amsterdam: Elsevier.

Pallis, C. A. & Spillane, J. B. (1957) A subacute progressive encephalopathy with mutism, hypokinesia, rigidity and myoclonus. *Q. Jl Med.*, **26**, 349.

Pampiglione, G. (1964) Prodromal phase of measles—some neurophysiological studies. *Br. med. J.*, **iv**, 1296.

Petsche, H., Schinko, H. & Seitelberger, F. (1961) Neuro-pathological studies on van Bogaert's subacute sclerosing leucoencephalitis. In *Encephalitides*, ed. van Bogaert, L., Radermecker, J., Hozay, J. & Lowenthal, A., pp. 353–85. Amsterdam: Elsevier.

Radermecker, J. (1949) Aspects électroencéphalographiques dans trois cas d'encéphalite subaiguë. *Acta neurol. belg.*, **49**, 222.

Radermecker, J. (1956) Systématique et électroencéphalographie des encéphalites et encéphalopathies. *Electroenceph. clin. Neurophysiol.*, Suppl. 5, 226.

Radermecker, J. & Poser, C. M. (1960) The significance of repetitive paroxysmal electroencephalographic patterns. *Wld Neurol.*, **1**, 422.

Rawls, W. E., Dyck, P. J., Klass, D. W., Greer, H. D. & Herrmann, E. C. (1966) Encephalitis associated with herpes simplex virus. *Ann. int. Med.*, **64**, 104.

Sever, J. L. & Zeman, W. (1968) Conference on measles virus and subacute sclerosing panencephalitis. *Neurology, Minneap.*, **18**, 2.

Storm van Leeuwen, W. (1964) Electroencephalographical and neurophysiological aspects of subacute sclerosing leucoencephalitis. *Folia psychiat. neurol. neurochir. neerl.*, **67**, 312.

Upton, A. & Gumpert, J. (1970) Electroencephalography in diagnosis of herpes simplex encephalitis. *Lancet*, **i**, 650.

Vincent, D., Cohadon, S., Loiseau, P. & Fontanges, X. (1969). L'électro-encéphalogramme des encéphalites aiguës nécrosantes. *Rev. neurol.*, **120**, 466.

6

Treatment of Viral Encephalitis

L. S. ILLIS

In the last 10 years or so there has been an increasing recognition and diagnosis of viral encephalitis as being due to specific viruses, and specific syndromes (such as herpes simplex encephalitis) have been delineated. Over the same period of time the part played by viruses in so-called 'degenerative' disease of the central nervous system has progressively assumed more importance. Treatment of these conditions remains controversial. In this chapter the main discussion is about the types of encephalitis mentioned elsewhere in this book, and particularly herpes simplex encephalitis, which is probably the commonest form of severe sporadic encephalitis of temperate countries.

The problems encountered in the management of encephalitis are those which may arise in any acute and severe involvement of the central nervous system and will not be dealt with here (see page 9).

If one outlines the process of virus infection in a highly simplified way and purely from the point of view of treatment, there are two main series of events.

Virus infection is followed by replication and spread of virus, viraemia and the development of the clinical picture (Fig. 5). In response to virus infection are host defence mechanisms (which may themselves add to the clinical picture). Host defences include

the production of interferon, which is an early reaction, the
production of antibody, which is relatively delayed, and the

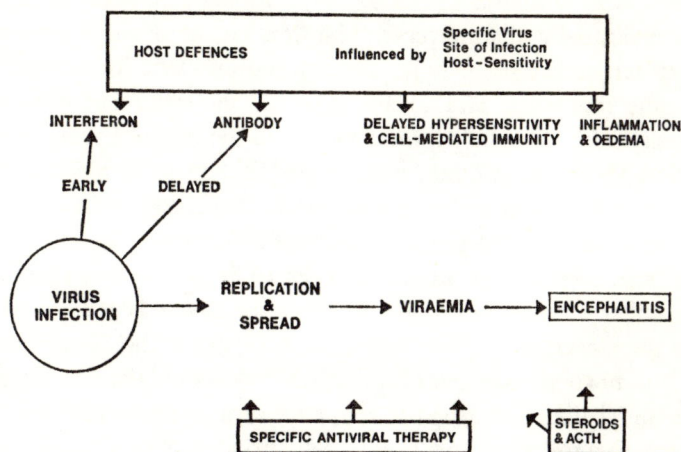

Fig. 5. The development of the clinical picture in virus infection.

development of delayed hypersensitivity and cell-mediated immunity. During this series inflammation develops. These host
defences are influenced by the specific virus and its site of infection, by host-sensitivity, and by immunosuppressive agents.
These events are interdependent and dictate the success or
failure of treatment. From a clinical point of view, specific antiviral therapy must be set against this background.

ANTIVIRAL AGENTS

Antiviral agents are compounds which prevent or inhibit the
replication of virus, as opposed to non-specific compounds which
produce their effect by altering the host response to infection. The
antiviral agents may act outside the cell (e.g. neutralizing antibody
or isoquinoline derivatives), at the cell surface (e.g. amantadine),

or inside the cell. Many of these antiviral agents are derived from cancer chemotherapy.

It has been said, with perhaps undue pessimism, that the progress of antiviral chemotherapy has been marked more by disappointment than success. The time course of virus infection is so rapid that there is hardly any time present for instituting specific treatment, and in any case specific treatment does not usually exist. This holds, for example, in rabies, poliomyelitis and yellow fever. In addition, virus multiplication takes place within the cell and it is quite likely that any therapeutic measure directed at the virus will also produce undesirable or disastrous effects on the host. This pessimism is, however, unfounded, since there are a number of virus infections in which the course is protracted or the manifestation of the disease is such that if the chemotherapeutic substance was available it would be easy to introduce during the initial illness and before the more serious phase had started. Some chemotherapeutic agents are available and, although the progress of antiviral chemotherapy does not match the rapid development of antibacterial therapy, there is clear indication of the possibilities for treatment of some virus diseases of the nervous system, including, potentially, the 'slow virus' infections.

Thiosemicarbazones
Thiosemicarbazones were first synthesized in 1895 but were not used as chemotherapeutic substances until the 1940s when they were developed for the treatment of tuberculosis. Their antiviral properties were discovered more or less by accident when they were tested against vaccinia virus. The compound most used in man is methisazone and this has been shown to be effective in the prophylaxis of smallpox (Bauer et al. 1963). This was the first demonstration of a drug effective in virus disease in man.

The antiviral thiosemicarbazones act intracellularly but although they may inhibit the multiplication of herpes virus in some cell systems, the amount of inhibition of herpes simplex is too small to be of any therapeutic value.

Amantadine

Amantadine hydrochloride will inhibit some influenzal viruses in culture, but the protective effect is slight. Several prophylactic trials of amantadine have been carried out with conflicting results. For example, in a double-blind trial in volunteers infected with influenza A2 virus, there was no clinical or laboratory evidence of antiviral effect (Tyrrell et al. 1965). A field trial investigating the spread of infection to household contacts, however, was effective with A2 virus (Galbraith et al. 1969).

One of the most important recent developments in neurology is the recognition that some of the so-called degenerative diseases of the nervous system are in fact due to transmissible agents. The reports of treatment of such conditions with antiviral compounds have therefore been of great interest. A few cases of Jakob–Creutzfeldt disease have been described with apparently successful treatment using amantadine. Braham (1971) described a single case with improvement after treatment. Unfortunately, it was impossible to obtain histological proof of the diagnosis. Sanders and Dunn (1973) reported 2 cases with partial remission in 1 case, and cure in the second. However, the diagnosis in the second case is doubtful (see page 154).

These results are encouraging, but remain uncertain. A personal case of Jakob–Creutzfeldt disease was treated with amantadine 600 mg per day. The patient had been admitted in coma; at the end of one week of treatment there was some clinical improvement in that the patient now responded to her name. There was no definite change in the electroencephalogram. Further treatment with cytarabine, 100 mg intravenously for 5 days produced no change, and the patient subsequently progressively deteriorated and died. (The only other point of note about this case is that cytomegalo-virus titre in the blood rose from 320 to 2560—this was presumably an opportunistic infection.)

Subacute sclerosing panencephalitis has been treated with purine and pyrimidine derivatives (see page 94) with poor results. A personal case treated with amantadine (300 mg per day) showed no clinical or definite electroencephalographic changes.

Guanidine

Guanidine inhibits the replication of sensitive viruses at levels which do not interfere with cellular metabolism. Viruses sensitive to guanidine include all 3 types of polio virus, coxsackie virus and ECHO virus. These usually cause a meningeal illness and only occasionally an encephalitis. Herpes simplex and herpes B virus are not inhibited by guanidine and it is doubtful if this drug has any major part to play in human therapy.

Purines and pyrimidines

Since DNA and RNA consist of purine and pyrimidine bases, these compounds and their analogues and antagonists form a logical approach to the problem of antiviral therapy.

Purines Purines have so far been disappointing. The only report of treatment in humans is that of 8 patients with Dawson's inclusion body encephalitis (subacute sclerosing panencephalitis; SSPE) who were given a purine derivative, 8-azaguanine (Hall et al. 1968). There was no clinical improvement.

Pyrimidines Pyrimidines have been used extensively against virus infection in man, nearly always in DNA virus infections (for a comprehensive list see Schabel & Montgomery 1972). The clinical reports of pyrimidines in RNA virus infections are few and unconvincing. For example, the use of 5 'bromo-2'-deoxyuridine (BUDR) in SSPE (see Freeman 1969), shows no definite evidence of benefit. The poor results with 8-azaguanine and BUDR in SSPE are not surprising, since these drugs specifically interfere with DNA metabolism and are not primarily effective against RNA viruses. BUDR was originally used at a time when SSPE was thought possibly to be due to a DNA virus and some improvement was noted in 2 cases.

Pyrimidines in DNA virus infections Good response to treatment has been demonstrated in a variety of human infections. These include warts, smallpox, vaccinia, varicella and zoster, and cytomegalus infection in the newborn.

94

In herpes simplex infections, there is undoubted benefit in the treatment of cutaneous, conjunctival, oral and genital herpes infections with idoxuridine (see Juel-Jensen & MacCallum 1972). In herpes simplex encephalitis, however, the role of idoxuridine and of Ara-C (cytarabine cytosine arabinoside $= 1$-β-D-arabino-furanosyl derivative of cytosine) is not yet established, and is still under investigation.

These compounds may act as mutagens or teratogens, and also have a possible carcinogenic action since they may be incorporated into the DNA molecule. They should therefore be used with caution.

Idoxuridine

Idoxuridine (IDU) is a thymidine analogue with an iodine atom replacing the 4-methyl group. Virus replication is inhibited by competitive blocking of the uptake of thymidine into the DNA molecule. IDU is incorporated in place of thymidine and an aberrant DNA molecule is formed.

The first clinical use of IDU was in the treatment of neoplastic disease, where it was considered to be ineffective. It was observed, however, that cancer patients undergoing treatment with IDU were not developing positive reactions with smallpox vaccine and this suggested that IDU might be useful in treating systemic DNA viral infections.

Intravenous infusion of IDU at a dosage of 100–120 mg/kg over a period of 2 to 3 hours daily for 5 to 6 days gives significant blood levels for approximately 4 hours. Toxic effects are related to the capacity of the drug to inhibit rapidly proliferating cells (Calabresi 1963). Administration of ^{125}I-idoxuridine confirmed that tissues are exposed to the intact drug for only short periods of time. The urinary excretion of the drug is rapid and about half the dose is likely to be excreted within 13 hours. In an attempt to see whether there was any uptake into the brain after the drug had been administered by the intravenous route, Breeden et al. (1966) administered radioactive IDU in a case of necrotizing temporal lobe encephalitis due to herpes simplex. Brain scan failed to show uptake. This does not necessarily indicate failure to enter the brain, since the drug concentration may have been inadequate to be demonstrated on scanning. Experimental distribution of radioactive-labelled IDU in plasma and cerebrospinal fluid of dogs shows a CSF:plasma ratio of 0·1:1. There was no evidence of any significant quantity of IDU reaching the cerebrospinal fluid after intravenous injection. Even when IDU is given directly into the cerebrospinal fluid there is rapid disappearance of the drug with concomitant appearance of iodouracil and iodine, suggesting that there is a rapid metabolism (Clarkson et al. 1967). Buckley and MacCallum (1967) measured the lumbar cerebrospinal fluid levels of IDU two hours after intra-arterial administration in a patient with herpes simplex encephalitis. Less than 20 μg/ml was found to be present. Intrathecal idoxuridine in rabbits infected with herpes simplex produced no beneficial effect (Kaufman 1963).

It would seem that IDU is too rapidly metabolized when injected intravenously or into the cerebrospinal fluid to have any real effect in encephalitis. However, there is no definite reason why the effectiveness of a drug should be equated with the level it attains in the cerebrospinal fluid and there have been many reports of cases in which idoxuridine treatment has appeared to be of benefit. Tomlinson and MacCallum (1973) showed a therapeutic effect in experimental herpes simplex encephalitis in guinea pigs, using IDU.

The first reports of successful treatment with IDU in herpes simplex encephalitis were those of Breeden et al. (1966) and Evans et al (1967). The potential benefit likely to be obtained remains, however, controversial. Analysis of treated cases from the literature and from personal experience (Illis & Merry 1972; Illis & Gostling 1972) indicated that the mortality rate falls from about 70% for untreated herpes simplex encephalitis (HSE) (overall mortality, Table 10) to 31%.

Many of the treated cases were left with grave neurological or mental sequelae. The clinical impression was that the earlier the patients were treated, the better the chance of survival, but analysis of the cases indicated that even when treatment was started several weeks after the onset of the illness, there was a good chance

TABLE 10

MORTALITY RATE IN HERPES SIMPLEX
ENCEPHALITIS

Reference	Mortality rate (%)
Ross & Stevenson 1961	13
Leider et al. 1965	25
Rawls et al. 1966	100
Miller et al. 1966	50
Olson et al. 1967	70
Dudgeon 1970	90
Overall mortality of 188 untreated cases	70

After Illis & Gostling 1972.

of survival. The treated patients who died tended to be older than those who survived following treatment, but the numbers were too small to permit any firm conclusion to be drawn. Nevertheless, the mortality rate by decades of untreated cases (Table 11) indicates that the mortality varies little with age, and there remains, therefore, a strong impression that the chances of treatment with IDU being of benefit is greater in patients under the age of fifty years (Illis & Merry 1972). Similarly, Juel-Jensen and

TABLE 11

MORTALITY RATE BY AGE OF UNTREATED CASES
OF HERPES SIMPLEX ENCEPHALITIS

Age	Mortality rate (%)
Under 10	68
11–20	56
21–30	83
31–40	50
41–50	70
51–60	77
61–70	75
71–80	83
Overall mortality	70

After Illis & Gostling 1972.

97

MacCallum (1972) found that older patients were more likely to die or survive with gross defects, and noted that 38% mortality occurred in the treated cases against their estimate of 55% mortality in the untreated group.

Toxic effects are common (Illis & Merry 1972) and include bone marrow depression (anaemia, leucopenia, thrombocytopenia), abnormal liver function tests, alopecia, stomatitis and glossitis, jaundice, gastrointestinal haemorrhage and diarrhoea in that order of frequency (Table 12). These toxic effects are reversible and no

TABLE 12

TOXIC EFFECTS OF IDOXURIDINE TREATMENT
IN 29 PATIENTS WITH HERPES SIMPLEX
ENCEPHALITIS

Toxic effects	No. of patients
Bone marrow depression (anaemia, leucopenia, thrombocytopenia)	16
Abnormal liver function tests	10
Alopecia	8
Stomatitis and glossitis	5
Jaundice	2
Gastrointestinal haemorrhage	1
Diarrhoea	1
No toxic effect	10

After Illis & Merry 1972.

deaths have been definitely attributable to the effects of IDU. The onset of marrow depression is usually about the seventh day (Geary 1973) and this is commonly the first sign of toxicity with thrombocytopaenia as an early manifestation.

Cytarabine
Cytarabine was developed originally as an anti-tumour agent and was found to be effective against DNA viruses in cell culture. A comparative study of experimental herpes simplex encephalitis in rabbits showed cytarabine to be superior to idoxuridine (Hall et al. 1968). Tomlinson and MacCallum (1973) reported work on guinea pigs with experimental herpes simplex encephalitis. They showed

that idoxuridine was therapeutic 'even when given on day 4 to pigs expected to die on days 5–7', but the effect was erratic. Cytarabine, on the other hand, was without effect. Their conclusion was that from the evidence of animal models the case for chemotherapy of herpes encephalitis was not proven. Similarly Rappel (1973), after an extensive survey of the management of reported cases, stated 'No treatment seems to be preferable to others'.

One problem is that there is no suitable laboratory model for herpes simplex encephalitis comparable to the clinical course in humans, and for this reason it is very difficult to assess the relative importance of experimental findings in relation to clinical experience. For example, in most animal work there is experimental infection with a sudden massive dose of virus which almost certainly does not occur in human infection.

The mode of action of cytarabine is not known, but it is thought either to become incorporated into DNA and so form an abnormal molecule or to inhibit the synthesis of DNA. Unlike idoxuridine, cytarabine has an immunosuppressive action (see Juel-Jensen & MacCallum 1972), but definite advantages of this drug are that it is widely used in the treatment of leukaemia and is therefore freely available; the side effects are probably less frequent than those reported in idoxuridine, and cytarabine is soluble in water and is easily prepared.

As with idoxuridine, side effects are common, and of a similar nature. Haematological effects are apparently variable and unpredictable. For instance, Geary (1973) reports striking megaloblastosis developing within hours as a feature of treatment, but quotes Juel-Jensen (1971, cited by Geary 1973) as reporting no signs of marrow depression. Pyrimidine analogues inhibit nucleic acid synthesis, or form an aberrant molecule, and damages to tissues with a high cell division rate are bound to be adversely affected.

Although disturbance of marrow function occurs, most experience has been in patients suffering malignant disease and Juel-Jensen and MacCallum (1972) find the drug to be relatively non-toxic in patients with normal marrow. Geary (1973) stresses the importance of marrow aspiration in assessing myeloid depression, since the peripheral blood count may be misleading, and cites a patient with a completely aplastic marrow after 6 days of treatment with Ara-C (cytarabine). In general, side effects of cytarabine include megaloblastosis, thrombocytopenia, pancytopenia, aplastic anaemia, immunosuppression, gastrointestinal disturbance, renal damage, hepatic damage, rashes and possibly chromosomal changes.

Interferon

A completely different approach to the problem of antiviral treatment stems from the phenomenon of viral interference, that is the suppression of replication of one virus by another virus. Virus interference has been observed repeatedly in plant virus diseases since the 1920s and probably dates back even further, since Jenner observed that herpes may prevent the development of vaccinia lesions. The production of interferon and the response appears to be a widespread biological phenomenon (Friedman & Buckler 1972). The interfering substance which is a result of virus infection is produced in the cell and was labelled 'interferon' by Isaacs and Lindenmann (1957). Interference is present early in infection, during the stage of viraemia, and before the occurrence of pathological changes. It appears, therefore, to be a factor in the host's natural cellular defence mechanisms. Measurable antibody is delayed in comparison and inhibits subsequent viral activity (e.g. dissemination and re-infection). Interferon is itself not antiviral but probably inhibits viral replication by stimulating the synthesis of a cellular protein which inhibits some viral function. In addition, interferon may inhibit cell growth and enhance phagocyte activity (Stewart et al. 1973). An interesting and potentially important point therapeutically is that the immune system and the interferon system appear to be intimately linked and sensitized cells may even initiate interferon production (see Grossberg 1972). The effect of immunosuppressive agents (including steroids) on this system is not known.

Unfortunately, although interferon has a wide spectrum of antiviral activity, its use is limited. There have been few encouraging reports of the beneficial effects of interferon in human virus infections. Successful examples include the use of large doses of interferon in rhinovirus type 4 infection (Merigan et al. 1973) and against vaccinia, influenza and cytomegalovirus (see Grossberg 1972 for references). Obvious difficulties include the species-specificity problem, and the production of sufficient quantities of human interferon is at present technically almost unsurmountable. Another possibility for the use of interferon is to employ inducers which stimulate interferon production, but in established infections it is unlikely that interferon will save virus infected cells.

The effect of interferon or of interferon inducers in herpes simplex encephalitis is not known. Interferon is not produced by and does not seem to have any effect upon the development of some of the 'slow' infections of the nervous system (see page 195).

Transfer factor and cell-mediated immunity
The use of transfer factor in virus diseases is hardly outside the experimental stage, and it may appear surprising to devote much time to discussion of its possible use. However, this method of treatment is of potential importance and a short review is therefore justifiable.

The immune response consists of antibody formation and a cell-mediated component (cellular mediated immunity or CMI). Persistent infections by many organisms including viruses may be associated with defective or abnormal CMI, although antibody is not abnormal. Cellular immunity in man may be transferred by injection of non-sensitive individuals with an extract of leucocytes from sensitive patients. Although the exact physicochem ica entities are not known, the transfer activity is associated with a low molecular weight substance, which is remarkably resistant to freezing, thawing, trypsin, DNAase and RNAase. It is not analogous to any known immunoglobulin and it is not itself immunogenic. Transfer factor as isolated and used at present may in fact contain more than one active principle. The CMI response concerns the destruction or damage of host cells which have acquired a new antigen (or tumour cells). The mechanism of the transfer and the response is not clear, but one possibility is that transfer factor activates recipient's lymphocytes to produce antigen-specific cells (and possibly interferon).

Depressed, absent or abnormal cell-mediated immunity occurs in various conditions and it may be that the disease states are in fact due to the CMI deficiency. If this is so transfer factor would relieve the condition. Transfer factor has been used in man, e.g. in disseminated vaccinia (Kempe 1960) and in candidiasis (Schulkind et al. 1972; Valdimarsson et al. 1972), with good effect. Valdimarsson et al. (1974) have treated 8 SSPE patients with transfer factor, reasoning that the principal immunological abnormality in SSPE is an unduly high antibody titre with blocking of the cellular immune response. Immunological changes have been demonstrated but, so far, no definite clinical improvement has been observed.

CMI against a virus may be both protective and damaging. In some forms of virus infection, such as lymphocytic choriomeningitis, CMI may be more damaging than the virus itself, whereas in other infections, e.g. poliomyelitis, CMI is protective. A deficient CMI may aggravate the dissemination of viral infection. It is possible that cell-mediated responses may be more important than antibodies in resistance to some viral infections, and although understanding of this sort of response is poor, there is potentially a wide application in viral therapy (Mims 1973). A further possibility is that the progressive course seen, for example, in SSPE, is not due, or not only due, to virus replication and cell death, but is possibly related to the very high levels of measles antibody in serum and cerebrospinal fluid.

A personal case of SSPE had an anti-measles titre of 16 000. Immunofluorescent examination of blood (Professor G. T. Stevenson) showed surface Ig on all white cells (granulocytes and lymphocytes). This could represent antibody on viral antigens and this may perhaps inhibit function—possibly CMI. If this is so, then there is a case for immunosuppression in order to lower the antibody resistance. The CMI component would also be affected, but probably to a lesser degree. The chances of secondary infection, of course, would be very high and the dangers of immunosuppression would be great. The patient has now been under treatment with transfer factor by Dr H. Valdimarsson for eight months. She has been given 15 injections of transfer factor prepared from approximately 39 pints of blood, and has had plasmaphoresis on 3 occasions. Initially there was a fall in measles antibody in serum and CSF. Although the rate of fall has not been maintained, antibodies remain at a relatively low level for SSPE and have remained stable for about 3 months. During the first 2 months her physical condition remained stable but with a subsequent deterioration with incontinence of urine and inability to walk unsupported. After the third plasmaphoresis there was striking improvement lasting for one week and followed again by physical deterioration. There has been no definite intellectual deterioration. Before treatment with transfer factor was started the clinical picture was of progressive deterioration.

Steroids and ACTH

The use of ACTH and steroids in the treatment of severe infection remains, at the least, controversial. In the case of bacterial infections results have been investigated repeatedly and a certain amount of scepticism remains. In viral infections evaluation has been more difficult, partly because of the frequent publication of isolated cases and partly because individual physicians see only relatively few cases so that it is difficult to arrive at a conclusive view of the value of personally treated cases. Steroids in vitro enhance virus replication (Kilbourne & Horsfall 1951) and suppress the synthesis and action of interferon (Kilbourne et al. 1961). Intraperitoneal injection of polio virus in animals treated with steroids (Schwartzman 1954) produces paralysis, but no paralysis is produced if the injection is into animals not treated with steroids. The local application of steroids to patients with herpes zoster and herpes simplex infections may result in severe exacerbation. Tokumaru (1968) inoculated guinea pigs intracerebrally with herpes simplex virus and observed the effect on survival of various types of treatment. Idoxuridine and interferon given for 5 days each showed a definite therapeutic effect. Hydrocortisone had no effect given as a 5-day course or as a single dose. Prednisolone may increase the risks of secondary or intercurrent infection in patients with a severe neutropenia such as may be induced by idoxuridine or cytarabine. Corticosteroids are not only immunosuppressive in their own right but may potentiate other immunosuppressive drugs. The long-term use of corticosteroids in high dosage is associated with a high complication rate and an appreciable mortality. Complications include peptic ulceration, massive infection, hypertension, increased morbidity from diabetes mellitus, osteoporosis, muscular wasting and eye complications including glaucoma and cataract. Patients on treatment with immunosuppressive agents, including steroids, are at particular risk from infection. This is seen for example in transplant patients where reduced resistance to herpes simplex, cytomegalovirus and fungi is common and is now the main cause of death after organ transplants (Lessof 1973). Juel-Jensen and MacCallum (1972) state that they 'are not convinced that it may not help to facilitate the spread of virus'. Virus infections (other than slow virus) of the central nervous system are usually associated with an inflammatory reaction which may be the expression of antibody response. However, in immunosuppressed hosts there is either no antibody formation or a deficient response and the pathological changes of degenerative lesions resemble the changes observed in slow virus infections of the scrapie–kuru type (see pages 122, 129). Extended use of steroids may produce fluid retention and indeed benign intracranial hypertension may follow.

Boe et al. (1965) described a retrospective study (in Norway) of the effect of corticosteroid treatment in 346 patients suffering from acute meningoencephalitis in which the aetiological agents were not stated. Of these, 91 cases had a post-infectious encephalitis, 153 were not post-infectious, and 102 patients had an encephalitis of uncertain type. In all three groups the mortality rates were higher in the corticosteroid group. There were 106 cases who were comatose during the acute stage of the illness and it is patients in this group who are perhaps more likely to receive steroid therapy. The authors therefore analysed this group separately. Again the results indicated a higher mortality in the treated (69·2%) than in the non-treated group (58·2%). The frequency of neurological sequelae was also higher in the corticosteroid treated group of patients (73% : 27·6%). It is true that these findings are subject to the usual strictures of retrospective studies. Nevertheless, the analysis was carefully done and the findings must be accepted as significant.

There have been several quite conflicting reports of the effect of steroids. Page et al. (1967) reported 2 patients with herpes simplex encephalitis who were treated with dexamethasone and both died. The authors felt that steroids were contraindicated in this condition. More recently, however, Upton et al. (1971) described 2 cases in which treatment with dexamethasone was followed by improvement. These authors concluded that steroids should be used in emergency treatment in this condition while further diagnostic measures are taken. Corticosteroids, however, act too slowly to be of much benefit in the moribund patient and there are more rapid procedures to reduce cerebral oedema (see page 107). Longson and Beswick (1971) contested the report of Upton et al. (1971) and pointed out that steroids may inhibit the production of interferon and of viral antibody, increase viral virulence and, particularly in herpes simplex infections, lead to a worsening of disease with occasional disastrous results.

It appears therefore that there is much evidence suggesting that treatment with steroids may be positively harmful. However, in many virus diseases of the nervous system, symptoms appear at about the time of significant levels of antibody in the circulation. This suggests that the disease is in fact due in part to a hypersensitivity reaction to virus replication and not a direct toxic effect. If this is so then one would expect an immunosuppressive agent to be effective. Immunosuppressive agents (including steroids) produce many deleterious effects in experimental models but the results are not strictly applicable to man since most, if not all, experimental animals are infected by a sudden massive dose of virus and this almost certainly does not occur in human infection. Webb and Hall (1972) question whether the primary cytopathic effect or the allergic response is of greater importance in the *clinical* situation. They produce evidence to show that the allergic response may add to mortality and morbidity in virus disease. An organ such as the brain, confined by a rigid skeleton, is particularly vulnerable to anoxia and ischaemia and circulatory disturbance, which may occur secondary to inflammation. In clinical practice, as opposed to experimental models, a full allergic state is present and immunosuppressive treatment will do little to alter this at the levels usually given. But immunosuppressive treatment will produce an anti-inflammatory effect which may be of greater clinical importance than immunosuppression. In other words, the allergic response may of itself produce damaging results in virus disease. Webb and Hall's final sentence is worth quoting in this context: 'when a member of an orchestra gets a few bars out of time, his continued efforts are likely to result in a chaotic disharmony and he would serve the cause of music better if he kept quiet'.

In an attempt to clarify the position of steroid therapy in herpes simplex encephalitis, Illis and Merry (1972) analysed cases from the literature, and personal cases, in which details of therapy were known. Surprisingly enough only a small number of cases in the literature were reported with the details of therapy and it is likely that in fact many more cases are treated but, because of the often fatal outcome and the fact that these cases were usually reported in the pathological literature, therapy was considered palliative or symptomatic and so not mentioned. In the cases collected it was apparent that steroid or ACTH therapy could lower the mortality of herpes simplex encephalitis from 70% to 44%. There was no evidence that the quality of survival was affected by the use of these drugs.

In summary, there are numerous studies which demonstrate that steroids enhance viral replication and decrease interferon synthesis and have many other deletereous or potentially deletereous effects. In the clinical situation, as opposed to the experimental model, there is no sudden beginning and the patient presents with a developing or developed allergic state. At this time it is likely that one of the dangers to the patient's life is brain swelling and the effects of inflammation. At this time steroids may have a great part to play, not as immunosuppressive agents but as anti-inflammatory and anti-oedema agents. Clinical studies are conflicting and the use of steroids should therefore be judged at least partly on the individual patient's clinical state with particular reference to evidence of brain swelling and progressive deterioration. Steroids should not be given without antiviral agents when these are available. In the specific case of herpes simplex encephalitis, it is suggested that treatment should be given according to the system worked out by the herpes simplex working party (see Appendix, page 112).

DECOMPRESSION

Obvious swelling of the brain is a distinct feature of herpes simplex encephalitis, and brain slices usually show evidence of oedematous swollen cortex, with a loss of the normal distinction between cortex and white matter. It is likely that brain swelling is often the cause of death, and measures to combat cerebral oedema are, therefore, of paramount importance. This is particularly so in the early stages of management, in the severely ill patient, before antiviral drugs have started to produce any effect.

Hypertonic solutions
Intravenous hypertonic solutions will reduce cerebral oedema quickly. The most widely used are urea and mannitol and the agent of choice in most neurosurgical units is mannitol. Mannitol appears to act as effectively as urea but for longer periods and with no rebound in pressure after the treatment has stopped. A 20% solution is given intravenously over 30 minutes and repeated every 4 to 6 hours as necessary.

Hypothermia
Hypothermia is still occasionally used but although there is evidence of potential benefit from experimental studies, in that cerebral metabolism is reduced, and there is protection against anoxia, clinical experience is less rewarding. Hypothermia probably takes several hours to have any effect and is therefore of less practical use than other measures.

Hyperventilation

Hyperventilation assures adequate oxygenation, increased venous return and decreased jugular venous pressure. The brain volume is decreased and this procedure, which acts quickly, may occasionally be life-saving since a considerable fall in intracranial pressure may be produced. However, lowering $P\text{co}_2$ reduces cerebral blood flow and the overall result may therefore be disappointing. The place of controlled respiration is more important since this should ensure normal $P\text{co}_2$ and $P\text{o}_2$ so that obstruction or otherwise impaired respiration does not lead to a rising $P\text{co}_2$ and exacerbation of oedema.

Steroids

The first report of the beneficial action of steroids, in this context, was probably of patients suffering from stroke illnesses (Roberts 1958). In the situation of acute viral encephalitis (notably herpes simplex encephalitis) corticosteroids act too slowly to be of benefit in the moribund patient. Steroids have a marked effect on cell membranes and this stabilizing effect may account for the benefit seen in cerebral oedema. In addition, these drugs may reduce cerebrospinal fluid production (Weiss & Nulsen 1969). The drug used in neurological practice is dexamethasone, 14 or 16 mg/day in divided doses. Gastrointestinal haemorrhage is a definite risk (Langfitt 1973).

Surgical decompression

In the extremely ill patient with evidence of progressive deterioration and raised intracranial pressure the measures mentioned above may not be sufficient. In these cases surgical decompression should be considered.

In 1956 Dodge and Cure reported the first case in which the diagnosis of encephalitis with inclusion bodies was established during life by brain biopsy. Serial serological studies suggested that the causal agent was herpes simplex virus. This patient survived the acute illness and the authors concluded that survival during the acute phase was at least partly due to surgical decompression carried out on the fifth day after onset, at a time when there was clinical and radiological evidence of raised intracranial pressure. This was the first case in which surgical decompression was performed as part of the treatment and since that time several authors have drawn attention to the possible value of decompressive craniotomy in cases where there is evidence of raised intracranial pressure and progressive clinical deterioration. The mortality rate of patients treated in this way is in the region of 30% (Illis & Merry 1972), and this figure is considerably lower than the overall mortality of untreated cases. The figures are, of course, not strictly comparable since the cases selected for decompression were characterized by their progressive deterioration and by the evidence of raised intracranial pressure. In addition, some other cases were treated with idoxuridine as well as surgical decompression. Nevertheless it appears that decompressive craniotomy is of value in *selected* cases. Clearly it is only feasible when there is radiographic evidence of marked unilateral *temporal lobe* swelling, preferably non-dominant, causing a significant midline shift. Without a generous anterior temporal lobectomy it is very doubtful that the older operation of subtemporal decompression and leaving the dura open, has any real effect.

Other measures to combat cerebral oedema are indicated and where these fail, and the patient's clinical state progressively deteriorates, and where there is still evidence of raised intracranial pressure, decompressive craniotomy should be considered. Treatment with antiviral drugs is indicated at the same time.

TREATMENT OF HERPES SIMPLEX ENCEPHALITIS

Since 1966 when the first cases of herpes simplex encephalitis treated with idoxuridine were reported, there have been many accounts of the beneficial effect of idoxuridine and, more recently, and not unexpectedly, more frequent reports of the ill effects of idoxuridine. We are still unfortunately relatively ignorant of the natural history of the disease. Undoubtedly patients survive without the 'benefit' of treatment and some of these patients may make a full and uncomplicated recovery. We still do not know the precise mortality and morbidity rate for untreated cases although it seems likely that the overall mortality is of the order of 70%. We still do not know the mortality and morbidity of patients treated by different methods, though steps are being taken to remedy this deficiency via the *Archives of Neurology* (Johnson 1972) in the United States, and the Herpes Simplex Working Party in the UK. The issue is complicated by the difficulty in establishing diagnosis without cerebral biopsy and by the publication of numerous reports of small series or isolated cases which contribute only marginally to the problem of treatment.

The discussion of methods of treatment revolves around those drugs which are of potential benefit or about which there is some argument, and the use of decompression, either by medical means or by decompressive craniotomy.

The antiviral compounds which may be of benefit in this condition are idoxuridine and cytarabine. The effects of these drugs have been summarized above and it is clear that at the present time there is no general consensus as to which is preferable in the treatment of herpes simplex encephalitis. Some authors may advocate one as opposed to the other but the situation is not clear, as has, for example, been summarized by Rappel (1973): 'In the present state of knowledge no treatment seems to be preferable to the others'; and by Tomlinson and MacCallum (1973): 'The conclusion is that from the published evidence of animal models the case for chemotherapy of herpes encephalitis is, at best, not proven'. On the whole, however, the evidence suggests that cytarabine is probably superior. For example, Oxbury (1974) has 4 patients treated with idoxuridine of whom 3 died and 7 patients treated with cytarabine of whom only 1 died. However, most if not all the evidence in favour of cytarabine is from uncontrolled trials and isolated reports. More recent experience (Dennis et al. 1974) does not confirm antiviral benefit of this drug in systemic infections. A controlled trial is clearly desirable.

The position of steroids in the treatment of herpes simplex encephalitis remains problematical as has already been made clear in the preceeding section. It is easy to put forward an almost insurmountable case against the use of steroids in viral encephalitis. However, most of the evidence is based on animal models and these are not strictly comparable to the clinical state. Many workers have put forward an equally convincing case for the use of steroids in this condition.

The question of decompression is much easier to resolve since clearly if there is evidence on clinical grounds of raised intra-cranial pressure then the patient should be treated with medical decompressive procedures (as detailed above) and where there is radiographic evidence of swelling causing a significant shift of midline structures, temporal lobectomy should be carried out.

These conflicting views about treatment are of course no help to a clinician faced with an acute problem of herpes simplex encephalitis. For this reason the Herpes Simplex Encephalitis Working Party has been set up in this country and in Europe with the aim of producing a multi-centre double-blind trial. At the present time a protocol for a sequential study of dexamethasone with or without cytarabine has been put forward and I would suggest that cases in this country and Europe are referred to a member of the working party. Where it is not possible to refer cases in this way then the treatment suggested is 10 mg cytarabine in 0·5 ml/kg body weight daily for 5 days. This should be given by a single bolus intravenous injection every 24 hours. This dose of cytarabine will probably, if not invariably, depress bone marrow. The first manifestation is likely to be a drop in reticulocyte count and platelet count. An aplastic marrow may occur and in this case the drug should be stopped and anabolic androgen steroids (oxy-metholone, methenolone, dromostanolone, 2 mg/kg/day) may be of value in treatment (Sanchez-Medal et al. 1969).

Clearly, cases which are not referred to the multi-centre trial must be treated at the discretion of the physician in charge. If dexamethasone is given then the suggested dose is as follows:

a. Children up to 10 kg body weight
  1 mg/kg loading dose
  2 mg every 6 hours for 8 doses
  2 mg every 12 hours for 4 doses
b. Children over 10 kg, and for average adults of up to 70 kg
  10 mg loading dose

4 mg every 6 hours for 8 doses
4 mg every 12 hours for 4 doses

Treatment should be continued longer if necessary.

It should be stressed that there is still considerable doubt as to which type of treatment is likely to be most effective. This doubt is only likely to be resolved by the collection of a large number of cases and wherever possible cases should be referred to the Working Party on Herpes Encephalitis (see Appendix).

Post-encephalitic treatment

All the known viral encephalitides may leave sequelae in terms of motor and intellectual or emotional deficits. The incidence and severity of such residual disturbances varies greatly and depends not only on differing virulence of viruses but also on host susceptibility and on the age of the patient. Anticonvulsant drugs and treatment of post-encephalitic psychological problems may be necessary (see page 9).

APPENDIX:
WORKING PARTY ON HERPES ENCEPHALITIS

Dr L. A. Liversedge (*Chairman*), Manchester; Dr Maurice Longson (*Secretary*), Clinical Laboratories, Manchester Royal Infirmary, Manchester M13 9WL; Professor Hume Adams, Glasgow; Dr D. B. Brownell, Bristol; Dr P. H. Buxton, Liverpool; Dr T. H. Flewett, Birmingham; Dr L. S. Illis, Southampton; Dr B. E. Juel-Jensen, Oxford; Dr F. O. MacCallum, Oxford; Dr G. D. W. McKendrick, London; Mr J. Douglas Miller, Glasgow; Dr J. M. Oxbury, Oxford; Dr Marc Rappel, Brussels; Dr M. V. Salmon, Smethwick; Mr P. G. Smith, Oxford; Dr R. N. P. Sutton, London; Dr C. E. C. Wells, Cardiff; Dr I. M. S. Wilkinson, Cambridge; Dr Thomas C. Hall (corresponding member), USA.

REFERENCES

Bauer, D. J., St Vincent, L., Kempe, C. H. & Downie, A. W. (1963) Prophylactic treatment of smallpox contacts with *N*-methylisatin β-thiosemicarbazone. *Lancet*, **ii**, 494.

Treatment of viral encephalitis

Boe, J., Solberg, C. O. & Saeter, T. (1965) Corticosteroid treatment for acute meningo-encephalitis: a retrospective study of 346 cases. *Br. med. J.*, **i**, 1094.

Braham, J. (1971) Jakob-Creutzfeld disease: treatment by amantadine. *Br. med. J.*, **iv**, 212.

Breeden, C. J., Hall, T. C. & Tyler, H. R. (1966) Herpes simplex encephalitis treated with systemic 5-iodo-2′deoxyuridine. *Ann. intern Med.*, **65**, 1050.

Buckley, T. F. & MacCallum, F. O. (1967) Herpes simplex virus encephalitis treated with idoxuridine. *Br. med. J.*, **ii**, 419.

Calabresi, P. (1963) Current status of clinical investigation with 6-asauridine, 5-iodo-2′deoxyuridine and related derivatives. *Cancer Res.*, **23**, 1260.

Clarkson, D. R., Oppelt, W. W. & Byvoet, P. (1967) The fate of 5-iodo-2′deoxyuridine in plasma and cerebrospinal fluid of dogs. *J. Pharmac. exp. Ther.*, **157**, 581.

Dennis, D. T., Doberstyn, E. B., Awoke, S., Royer, G. L. & Renis, H. E. (1974) Failure of cytosine arabinoside in treating smallpox. *Lancet*, **ii**, 377.

Dodge, P. R. & Cure, C. W. (1956) Acute encephalitis with intranuclear cellular inclusions: A nonfatal case of probable herpetic etiology diagnosed by biopsy. *New Engl. J. Med.*, **255**, 849.

Dudgeon, J. A. (1970) Herpes simplex. In *Modern Trends in Medical Virology*, ed. Heath, R. B. & Waterson, A. P. London: Butterworths.

Evans, A. D., Gray, O. P., Miller, M. H., Verrier Jones, E. R., Weeks, R. D. & Wells, C. E. C. (1967) Herpes simplex encephalitis treated with intravenous idoxuridine. *Br. med. J.*, **ii**, 407.

Freeman, J. M. (1969) Treatment of Dawson's encephalitis with 5-bromo-2′-deoxyuridine. *Archs Neurol., Chicago*, **21**, 431.

Freidman R. M. & Buckler, C. E. (1972) Virus-induced interferons. In *Chemotherapy of Virus Diseases*, ed. Bauer, D. J. Oxford: Pergamon.

Galbraith, A. W., Oxford, J. S., Schild, G. C. & Watson, G. I. (1969) Protective effect of 1-adamantanamine hydrochloride on influenza A2 infections in the family environment. *Lancet*, **ii**, 1026.

Geary, C. G. (1973) Haematological complications of therapy with pyrimidine analogues. *Postgrad. med. J.*, **49**, 413.

Grossberg, S. E. (1972) The interferons and their inducers: molecular and therapeutic considerations. *New Engl. J. Med.*, **287**, 122.

Hall, T. C., Griffiths, J., Watters, G., Baringer, R. & Katz, S. (1968) Anti-viral studies with anti-tumour agents. *Pharmacology*, **10**, 171.

Illis, L. S. & Gostling, J. V. T. (1972) *Herpes Simplex Encephalitis*. Bristol: Scientechnica.

Illis, L. S. & Merry, R. T. G. (1972) Treatment of herpes simplex encephalitis. *J. R. Coll. Physns*, **7**, 34.

Isaacs, A. & Lindenmann, J. (1957) Virus interference. I. Interferon. *Proc. R. Soc., B*, **147**, 258.

Johnson, R. T. (1972) Treatment of herpes simplex virus encephalitis. *Archs Neurol., Chicago*, **27**, 97.

Juel-Jensen, B. E. & MacCallum, F. O. (1972) *Herpes Simplex, Varicella and Zoster*. London: Heinemann.

Kaufman, H. E. (1963) Chemotherapy of virus disease. *Chemotherapia,* **7,** 1.

Kempe, C. H. (1960) Studies on smallpox and complications of smallpox vaccination. *Pediatrics, Springfield,* **26,** 176.

Kilbourne, E. D. & Horsfall, F. L. (1951) Increased virus in eggs injected with cortisone. *Proc. Soc. exp. Biol. Med.,* **76,** 116.

Kilbourne, E. D., Smart, K. M. & Pokorny, B. A. (1961) Inhibition by cortisone of the synthesis and action of interferon. *Nature, Lond.,* **190,** 650.

Langfitt, T. W. (1973) Increased intracranial pressure. In *Neurological Surgery,* ed. Youmans, J. R. Philadelphia: Saunders.

Leider, W., Magoffin, R. L., Lennette, E. H. & Leonards, L. N. R. (1965) Herpes simplex virus encephalitis. *New Engl. J. Med.,* **273,** 341.

Lessof, M. H. (1973) Immunosuppressive drugs and their adverse effects. *Prescrib. J.,* **13,** 141.

Longson, M. & Beswick, T. S. L. (1971) Dexamethasone treatment in herpes simplex encephalitis. *Lancet,* **i,** 749.

Merigan, T. C., Reed, S. E., Hall, T. S. & Tyrell, D. A. J. (1973) Inhibition of respiratory virus infection by locally applied interferon. *Lancet,* **i,** 563.

Miller, J. K., Hesser, F. & Tomkins, V. N. (1966) Herpes simplex encephalitis. *Ann. intern. Med.,* **64,** 92.

Mims, C. (1973) The immune response to viral infection. *Br. J. Hosp. Med.,* **10,** 385.

Olson, L. C., Buescher, E. L., Artenstein, M. S. & Parkman, P. D. (1967) Herpes virus infections of the human central nervous system. *New Engl. J. Med.,* **277,** 1271.

Oxbury (1974) Personal communication.

Page, L. K., Tyler, H. R. & Shillito, J. (1967) Neurosurgical experiences with herpes simplex encephalitis. *J. Neurosurg.,* **27,** 346.

Rappel, M. (1973) The management of acute necrotizing encephalitis: a review of 369 cases. *Postgrad. med. J.,* **49,** 419.

Rawls, W. E., Dyck, P. J., Klass, D. W., Greer, H. D. & Herrmann, E. C. (1966) Encephalitis associated with herpes simplex virus. *Ann. intern. Med.,* **64,** 104.

Roberts, H. J. (1958) Supportive adrenocortical steroid therapy in acute and subacute cerebro-vascular accidents, with particular reference to brain-stem involvement. *J. Am. geriat. Soc.,* **6,** 686.

Ross, C. A. C. & Stevenson, J. (1961) Herpes simplex meningo-encephalitis. *Lancet,* **ii,** 682.

Sanchez-Medal, L., Gomez-Leal, A., Duarte, L. & Rico, M. G. (1969) Anabolic androgenic steroids in the treatment of acquired aplastic anaemia. *Blood,* **34,** 283.

Saunders, W. L. & Dunn, T. L. (1973) Creutzfeld-Jacob disease treated with amantadine. *J. Neurol. Neurosurg. Psychiat.,* **36,** 581.

Schabel, F. M. & Montgomery, J. A. (1972) Purines and pyrimidines.

In *Chemotherapy of Virus Diseases*, ed. Bauer, D. J. Oxford: Pergamon.

Schulkind, M. L., Adler, W. H., Altemeier, W. A. & Ayoub, E. M. (1972) Transfer factor in the treatment of a case of chronic mucocutaneous candidiasis. *Cell. Immunol.*, **3**, 606.

Schwartzman, G. (1954) New aspects of pathogenesis of experimental poliomyelitis. *J. Mt Sinai Hosp.*, **21**, 3.

Stewart, W. E., Declercq, E., de Somer, P., Berg, K., Ogburn, C. A. & Paucker, K. (1973) Antiviral and non-antiviral activity of highly purified interferon. *Nature, Lond.*, **246**, 141.

Tokumaru, T. (1968) The protective effect of different immunoglobulins against herpes encephalitis and skin infection in guinea-pigs. *Arch. ges. Virusforsch.*, **22**, 332.

Tomlinson, A. H. & MacCallum, F. O. (1973) Pyrimidine analogues in the treatment of experimental herpes infections. *Postgrad. med. J.*, **49**, 416.

Tyrrell, D. A. J., Bynoe, M. L. & Hoorn, B. (1965) Studies on the antiviral activity of 1-adamantanamine. *Br. J. exp. Path.*, **45**, 370.

Upton, A. R. M., Barwick, D. D. & Foster, J. B. (1971) Dexamethasone treatment in herpes simplex encephalitis. *Lancet*, **i**, 290.

Valdimarsson, H., Agnarsdottir, G. & Lachman, P. J. (1974) Cellular immunity in subacute sclerosing panencephalitis. *Proc. R. Soc. Med.*, **67**, 1125.

Valdimarsson, H., Wood, C. B. S., Hobbs, J. R. & Holt, P. J. L. (1972) Immunological features in a case of chronic granulomatous candidiasis and its treatment with transfer factor. *Clin. exp. Immunol.*, **11**, 151.

Webb, H. E. & Hall, J. G. (1972) An assessment of the role of the allergic response in the pathogenesis of viral diseases. *Symp. Soc. gen. Microbiol.*, **22**, 383

Weiss, M. H. & Nulsen, F. E. (1969) Cited by Langfitt (1973).

PART TWO

Transmissible and Degenerative Diseases of the Nervous System

7

Introduction: Subacute Spongiform Encephalopathy

J. HUME ADAMS

The second part of this book is devoted principally to a group of progressive degenerative diseases of the central nervous system which are best referred to as the subacute spongiform encephalopathies. Two of these occur spontaneously in man, kuru and Jakob–Creutzfeldt disease, and two in animals, scrapie in sheep and progressive encephalopathy in mink. Each of these diseases can be transmitted to other species by 'agents' which have remarkable physical and biological properties (Gajdusek 1972; Gibbs & Gajdusek 1972), but the pathogenesis of the spontaneously occurring disease remains obscure, with the possible exception of kuru, where cannibalism appears to have been the principal mode of transmission (Alpers 1969). Because of these 'agents', the subacute spongiform encephalopathies now tend to be classified as 'slow virus infections' but the propriety of this has been questioned (Daniel 1971).

The four diseases have very similar neuropathology, the principal feature being a progressive degeneration of grey matter characterized by varying degrees of neuronal loss, status spongiosus and a florid astrogliosis (Beck et al. 1969, 1970). The white matter may appear normal with most of the conventional histological techniques although if selective stains for the breakdown products of myelin are used, there is evidence of degeneration of myelin attributable to widespread neuronal degeneration. A remarkable feature is the absence of any conventional inflammatory response in the brain or meninges. The disease profiles, however, i.e. the distribution and severity of the neuropathological changes, vary widely both in the naturally occurring disease and between the naturally occurring and experimentally induced disease. Thus there are several subtypes of Jakob–Creutzfeldt disease (see Daniel 1972; Adams et al. 1974), while the selective degeneration of the cerebellar and hypothalamohypophysial systems which are conspicuous features in naturally occurring scrapie and kuru is not a feature of the experimentally induced diseases (Beck & Daniel 1965). In contrast, status spongiosus in grey matter in the experimentally induced disease always tends to exceed in intensity that seen in naturally occurring scrapie and kuru. One sometimes wonders, therefore, particularly in regard to scrapie which has been recognized for a much longer time than the other subacute spongiform encephalopathies, if there is a tendency to devote too much time and effort to the experimentally induced disease and too little to the natural disease. No one, however, would pretend to deny the vital importance of the nature of the 'agent', particularly since the recent report of possible person-to-person transmission of Jakob–Creutzfeldt disease by a corneal transplant (Duffy et al. 1974).

The discovery that kuru and, later, Jakob–Creutzfeldt disease could be transmitted to primates has been one of the most dramatic developments in degenerative disease of man in the course of the last two decades. Daniel (1971) has suggested that the induction of changes in the brains of animals inoculated with material from scrapie, kuru and Jakob–Creutzfeldt disease represents a new biological phenomenon. I agree with this entirely. There certainly appear to be some unique features in the subacute spongiform encephalopathies.

REFERENCES

Adams, J. H., Beck, E. & Shenkin, A. (1974) Creutzfeld–Jakob disease: further similarities with kuru. *J. Neurol. Neurosurg. Psychiat.*, 37, 195.
Alpers, M. (1969) Kuru: clinical and aetological aspects. In *Virus Diseases and the Nervous System*, ed. Whitty, C. W. M., Hughes, J. T.

& MacCallum, F. O., pp. 83–97. Oxford and Edinburgh: Blackwell Scientific.

Beck, E. & Daniel, P. M. (1965) Kuru and scrapie compared: are they examples of a system degeneration. *Slow, Latent and Temperate Virus Infections*, ed. Gajdusek, D. C., Gibbs, C. J. & Alpers, M. pp. 85–93. Monograph No. 2, US Department of Health, Education and Welfare.

Beck, E., Daniel, P. M., Gajdusek, D. C. & Gibbs, C. J., jun. (1969) Similarities and differences in the pattern of the pathological changes in scrapie, kuru, experimental kuru and subacute presenile polio-encephalopathy. In *Virus Diseases and the Nervous System*, ed. Whitty, C. W. M., Hughes, J. T. & MacCallum, F. O., pp. 107–120. Oxford and Edinburgh: Blackwell Scientific.

Beck, E., Daniel, P. M., Gajdusek, D. C. & Gibbs, C. J., jun. (1970) Subacute degenerations of brain transmissible to experimental animals: a neuropathological examination. *Proc. VIth int. Congr. Neuropath.*, 858.

Daniel, P. M. (1971) Transmissible degenerative diseases of the nervous system. *Proc. R. Soc. Med.*, 64, 787.

Daniel, P. M. (1972) Creutzfeldt-Jakob Disease. *J. clin. Path.*, 25, Suppl. 6, 97.

Duffy, P., Wolf, J., Collins, G., DeVoe, A. G., Streeten, B. & Cowen, D. (1974) Possible person-to-person transmission of Creutzfeldt-Jakob disease. *New Engl. J. Med.*, 290, 692.

Gajdusek, D. C. (1972) Spongiform virus encaphalopathies. *J. clin. Path.*, 25, Suppl. 6, 78.

Gibbs, C. J., jun. & Gajdusek, D. C. (1972) Isolation and characterisation of the subacute spongiform virus encephalopathies of man: kuru and Creutzfeldt–Jakob disease. *J. clin. Path.*, 25, Suppl. 6, 84.

8

Virus Infection and Degenerative Conditions of the Central Nervous System

I. ZLOTNIK

Conventional virus infections of the central nervous system are usually associated with an inflammatory reaction and only slow viruses of the scrapie–kuru type give rise to primary degeneration and astrogliosis without being preceded by inflammation (Zlotnik 1970; Porter 1972). In addition to the above two diametrically different viral effects, there is also a group of infections of the CNS which start as inflammatory conditions, but after an initial phase either develop a tendency to become subacute in character accompanied by degenerative and sclerotic changes or, after the cessation of the acute reaction, leave sequelae in the form of temporary or permanent damage to the CNS (Davis 1940; Noran & Baker 1945; Zlotnik 1972; Zlotnik et al. 1972a, b, 1973).

Immunity plays a major role in determining the type of lesion produced in a virus infection of the CNS. Whereas in immunologically competent hosts the perivascular inflammatory reaction is the expression of antibody response to viral infection, in immunosuppressed or immunodeficient hosts, there is no antibody formation and no inflammation, but the appearance of degenerative lesions and astrogliosis. It is worth mentioning that the above changes in immunosuppressed hosts resemble the neuronal, glial and spongy degeneration observed in slow virus infections of the scrapie–kuru type (Nathanson & Cole 1970; Zlotnik et al. 1970, 1971; Zlotnik 1972b; Zlotnik & Grant 1973).

Experimental work with attentuated or vaccine strains of some viruses showed that severe chronic or subacute degenerative changes in the CNS may follow very mild initial inflammatory reactions and that the subacute process may progress for a very long time, long after live virus could be isolated from the brain of the experimental animal (Zlotnik et al. 1972a, b, 1973). The advantage of such experimental models is the possibility of following up, step by step, the appearance and disappearance of inflammatory changes and the formation of subacute and degenerative lesions. It allows also the study of the incidence of subacute, or chronic lesions and, by using sufficiently large numbers of animals, it enables the assessment of the risk of sequelae, even after very long periods. Such studies proved that even an inapparent infection of mice with an avirulent strain of Semliki Forest virus (SFV) may give rise to a progressive encephalopathy two years later (Zlotnik et al. 1972b). Thus there might be a good case for the argument that multiple sclerosis is connected with measles virus infection in early life, in spite of the fact that the majority of children get measles and only a very small proportion of the human race develops multiple sclerosis (Brody 1972; Brody et al. 1972; Cathala & Brown 1972).

Finally it must be emphasized that astrocytic gliosis, often associated with degenerative conditions of the CNS, is not necessarily an expression of chronicity, and does not appear only in the absence of an inflammatory reaction. On the contrary, very severe astrocytic proliferation and hypertrophy almost invariably accompanies acute and peracute viral infections of the CNS such as rabies, measles and arbovirus of group A and B. In some diseases, such as experimental Venezuelan equine encephalitis (VEE) infection of hamsters, astrocytosis forms the only morphological change in the CNS of animals dying as a result of respiratory or peripheral inoculations (Zlotnik 1968b). Thus the rigid distinction between the various forms of virus infection must be reconsidered in view of the fact that under certain circumstances the same virus may give rise to an acute encephalitis leading to either death or complete recovery or, in the absence of immune responses, may cause a degenerative type of encephalitis similar morphologically to the effects of slow virus infection or, finally, if strains are attenuated, may initiate an acute reaction which will produce a persistent infection leading to subacute and sclerotic lesions in some hosts.

As a whole, the various degenerative conditions of the CNS where viral aetiology might be implicated can be divided into four distinct groups as follows: slow virus infections of the scrapie-kuru type (spongiform encephalopathies), subacute persistent virus infections, sequelae to acute virus infections and lastly disease of the central nervous system where a virus aetiology can be reasonably postulated, but is not yet proven.

SLOW VIRUS INFECTIONS
(SPONGIFORM ENCEPHALOPATHIES)

This group of diseases differs from all other viral infections of the CNS in that no antibodies have ever been demonstrated in patients or animals affected with any of these diseases. On post-mortem examination, no inflammatory changes have been seen in the CNS or any other organs, but astrogliosis and spongiform degeneration of the brain and occasionally also of the spinal cord form the main pathological changes. The natural disease begins invariably in a very insidious way and progresses slowly to a fatal conclusion (Field 1969; Zlotnik 1970; Daniel 1971; Gadjusek 1972a, b; Lampert et al. 1972). The infective agents can be demonstrated at various stages of these diseases in the brain and in a number of other organs, especially the spleen and lymph nodes. Four diseases belong to the group of spongiform encephalopathies, two of which are human degenerative conditions, kuru and Jakob–Creutzfeldt disease, and two of which affect only animals, scrapie and transmissible mink encephalopathy. Two of these diseases, kuru and scrapie, are believed to have a familial character and the susceptibility to these conditions appears to be determined by a single gene.

Virus infection and degenerative conditions

The viruses or the transmissible agents of the four spongiform encephalopathies have a large number of common physical, chemical and biological properties, while the clinical and pathological changes in the hosts have many similarities (Stamp et al. 1959; Marsh & Hanson 1969; Marsh et al. 1969b; Gibbs & Gajdusek 1972a). They all appear to be highly resistant to the action of heat, ultra-violet light, formalin and other chemicals (Pattison 1965; Zlotnik & Stamp 1965, 1966; Alper 1972). Although the shape of these agents is hitherto unknown, the size of the scrapie agent is smaller than 50 nm and most probably 25–35 nm. However, the most striking common feature of all the four agents is the type of pathological change in the CNS. Although lesions in naturally affected hosts may differ between the four diseases and are often confined only to certain focal parts of the brain (Zlotnik 1958a, 1962a), on transmission to susceptible animals of a different species a change may take place, the lesions becoming widespread and affecting many parts of the brain.

Scrapie is the best known disease of this group and has been most extensively studied. In the natural disease of sheep, lesions are invariably confined to subcortical centres and in some breeds of sheep such as Cheviots, there is mainly only neuronal vacuolation in the brain stem and midbrain without diffuse spongiform degeneration (Plate III/1). On transmission to sheep and goats the pattern of brain lesions remained unaltered irrespective of the number of passages carried out and whether inoculation of the scrapie agent was by a peripheral or the intracerebral route (Zlotnik 1958b, 1961, 1962a, b). However, whereas lesions became often less marked and widespread in Cheviot sheep, in inoculated goats changes were usually widespread and present not only in the brain stem and midbrain but also in the thalamus, corpus striatum and paraterminal body. In the brain of infected goats, it was quite usual to find, apart from the usual lesions seen in sheep such as neuronal degeneration, vacuolation and astrogliosis and spongy degeneration of many areas especially the thalamus and paraterminal body. The incubation period in experimental animals was often reduced on second passage to 5 to 6 months for Cheviot sheep and 7 to 9 months for goats.

When scrapie was transmitted from sheep or goats to albino mice, the incubation period varied on first passage from 7 to 18 months, but on second mouse to mouse transmission was reduced to 4 to 5 months and remained so for several passages (Chandler 1961; Zlotnik & Rennie 1962, 1963; Zlotnik 1965).

The transmission of scrapie to mice, either from sheep or from goats, caused a basic change in the properties of the transmissible agent. This change did not become obvious until the first mouse-to-mouse passage was carried out. Thus on first transmission of scrapie from sheep and goats, brain lesions remained confined to subcortical centres and, in addition to neuronal and astrocytic changes, spongy degeneration became very obvious. After the first mouse-to-mouse passage the lesions became predominantly spongiform and affected all regions of the brain, including the cerebral cortex (Plate III/2, 3). On the other hand, if mouse brain of the first sheep or goat passage was heated for 30 minutes at 100°C the ability of the lesions to spread to cortical regions was abolished and remained so for 2 passages (Zlotnik & Rennie 1967). Thus heating every second mouse-to-mouse passage assured a continuation of lesions confined to subcortical centres. On the other hand if two mouse passages were carried out without heating the inoculum, lesions spread to the cortex and further heating of the inoculum after 2 unheated passages had no effect. It appears therefore that the ability of the lesions to spread to the cortex had been transmitted from the mouse and this factor was thermolabile only on first passage; thereafter it withstood the action of heat in the form of boiling for half an hour and longer. Further evidence of the stability of the mouse-adapted scrapie is derived from experimental transmissions of mouse scrapie to sheep, goats, hamsters, rats and cynomolgus monkeys. The agent in t ese animals gave rise to mouse type of brain lesions with diffuse spongy degeneration in many regions including the cerebral cortex (Chandler & Fisher 1963; Zlotnik 1963, 1965, 1970; Zlotnik & Rennie 1965; Gibbs & Gajdusek 1972c). When brain material from sheep and goats affected with mouse-type scrapie was subinoculated again into sheep or goats, the lesions remained widespread in the cerebral cortex, without reverting to the original changes seen in sheep or goat scrapie (Plate IV/1).

Various experiments have shown that scrapie disease can be transmitted by contact from infected to susceptible animals. However, hitherto contact transmissions have been carried out from naturally affected sheep to sheep and goats, but no evidence is forthcoming to show contact transmission from experimentally infected sheep or goats to sheep and goats. On the other hand, mouse scrapie, originally an experimental disease, is readily transmissible by contact to other mice (Dickinson et al. 1964; Brotherston et al. 1968; Zlotnik 1968a).

Transmissible mink encephalopathy (TME) is the second animal disease caused by a slow virus or agent akin to scrapie. In a way this is an enigmatic condition, in that it is not clear whether it is a separate entity, or just scrapie accidentally adapted to mink. The disease made its appearance in the form of a spontaneous outbreak amongst farmed mink in the USA. The physical properties of the transmissible agent, such as resistance to heat and size, are similar to those of scrapie, but the brain lesions in naturally affected mink resemble mouse scrapie in that spongy degeneration is present throughout the brain including the cerebral cortex (Marsh & Hanson 1969; Marsh et al. 1969a, b). However, although scrapie has been transmitted experimentally to mink, there is no real evidence to prove that TME has been transmitted to mice.

Up to the present, TME has been transmitted from mink to mink, goats, one-day-old hamsters, albino ferrets, squirrel monkeys and rhesus monkeys (Zlotnik & Barlow 1967; Marsh et al. 1969a; Barlow 1972). The brain lesions in experimentally infected mink do not differ from those in mink naturally affected with TME. On the other hand, in experimentally infected goats with TME the disease differs both clinically and pathologically from mouse-adapted scrapie in goats; the clinical signs are different and TME is not invariably fatal for goats, while hitherto all goats affected with scrapie died. The most striking brain change in TME is spongy degeneration of the cortical and subcortical grey matter, accompanied by astrogliosis, with only occasional neuronal vacuolation in the brain stem, whereas in mouse scrapie transmitted to goats the lesions are predominantly subcortical with typical vacuolations of neurones and only focal spongy degeneration of the cerebral cortex (Plate IV/2). Thus in spite of the similarities between TME and scrapie it is impossible at this stage to postulate a common origin of the two diseases.

The agents of the two human transmissible encephalopathies, kuru and Jakob–Creutzfeldt disease (JCD), have a considerable number of common properties with scrapie, including filtrability, heat stability and resistance to various chemicals (Davis 1940; Gibbs & Gajdusek 1972a; Lampert et al. 1972). The agents of both kuru and JCD have been transmitted to chimpanzees and to various monkeys. On first transmission to chimpanzees, however, the incubation period for kuru was 14 to 39 months and for JCD only 11 to 16 months. On further chimpanzee-to-chimpanzee transmission there was a dramatic drop in the length of the incubation period to 10 to 18 months in kuru, but in JCD it was only slightly reduced to 10 to 14 months. A comparison between the pathological changes in the brains of patients with kuru and JCD shows that in kuru lesions are more pronounced in the cerebellum and in the subcortical brain centres such as the brain stem, corpus striatum, olives and thalamus than in the cerebral cortex. The pathological changes consist of neuronal degeneration, cytoplasmic vacuolation, excessive lipochrome content, neuronophagia, astrogliosis, occasional demyelination of corticospinal and spinocerebellar tracts and anisotropic plaque-like bodies in the cerebellum. In Jakob–Creutzfeldt disease, on the other hand, there is status spongiosus of the grey matter of the cerebral cortex, variable loss of nerve cells, neuronal degeneration, neuronophagia and astrogliosis (Plates IV/3, V/1). Similar changes can be seen also in the cerebellum and in subcortical centres and, while myelin changes can be observed in the pyramidal tracts in the spinal cord, there is occasionally also degeneration of anterior horns (Field 1969; Daniel 1971, 1972; Lampert et al. 1972). In the chimpanzee, however, infected either with kuru or with JCD there is a marked increase in the intensity and spread of brain lesions. Especially severe status spongiosus of the cerebral hemi-

PLATE III

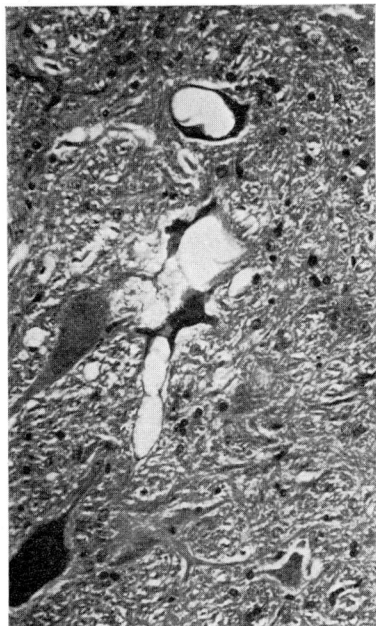

Fig. 1. Severe neuronal vacuolation in the medulla of sheep affected with scrapie.

Haematoxylin and eosin. × 200

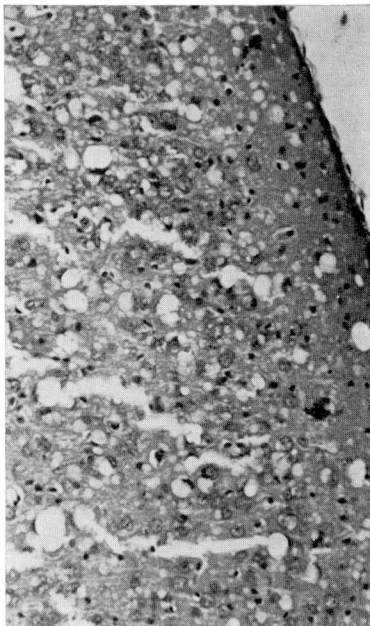

Fig. 2. Spongy degeneration of the cerebral cortex of mice infected with scrapie.

Haematoxylin and eosin. × 200

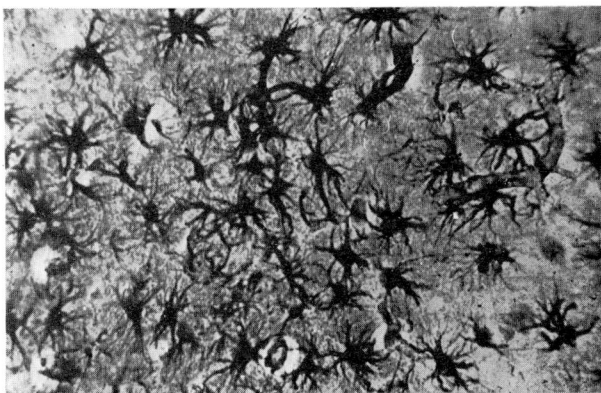

Fig. 3. Astrocytosis in the hippocampus of mice infected with scrapie.

Cajal. × 200

PLATE IV

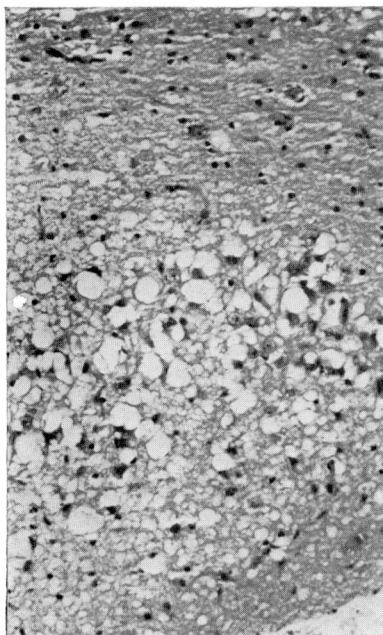

Fig. 1. Spongy degeneration of the cerebral cortex of goats infected with mouse scrapie.

Haematoxylin and eosin. × 200

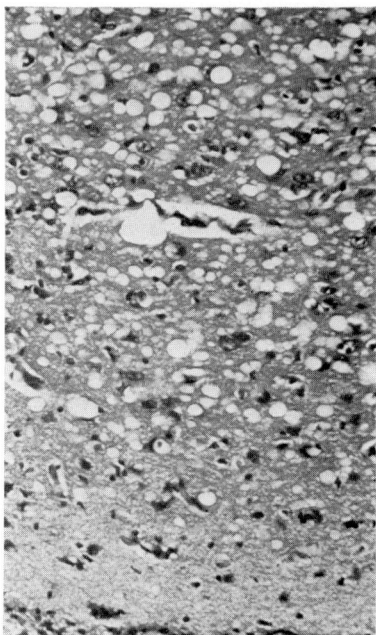

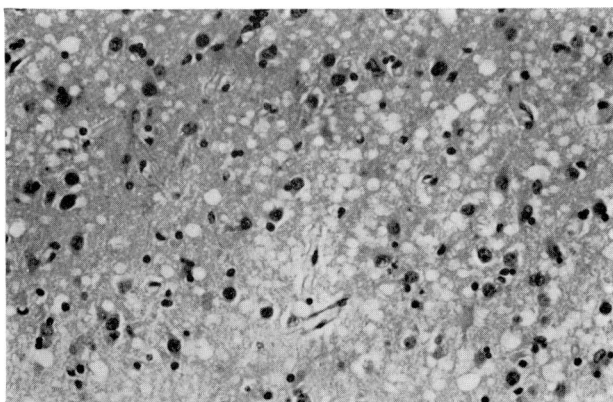

Fig. 2. Spongy degeneration of the cerebral cortex of goats infected with transmissible mink encephalopathy.

Haematoxylin and eosin. × 200

Fig. 3. Spongy degeneration of the human cerebral cortex in Jakob–Creutzfeldt disease.

Haematoxylin and eosin. × 200

spheres became apparent in chimpanzees infected with either of the diseases. In addition there was great loss of neurones and a notable increase in the number of hypertrophied astrocytes. Spongy degeneration was also a feature of the cerebellar cortex, but not of the same degree and extent as in the cerebral cortex. It is significant that the brain lesions in chimpanzees affected with either experimental kuru or Jakob–Creutzfeldt disease resemble those of mouse scrapie, TME in mink and in goats and mouse-passaged scrapie in hamsters, rats, monkeys, sheep and goats. However, at no time was there a similar spread of lesions to the cerebral cortex in natural scrapie of sheep or in sheep or goats inoculated with brain material from scrapie sheep or scrapie material that has been passaged several times either in sheep or in goats (Zlotnik 1958b, 1961, 1970).

It appears, therefore, that the morphological picture of the brain lesions, lack of antibody response, transmissibility and change in the pattern of brain lesions on transmission, are common factors for the four transmissible spongiform encephalopathies. It is rather disturbing that mice proved beyond a doubt to be susceptible to scrapie only and confirmation of the reports that TME and kuru have been transmitted to mice would be of special value in order to show a definite link between these diseases (Field 1968; Barlow 1972). Nevertheless the possibility of a common origin of the four encephalopathies in a very distant past cannot be excluded, especially as it is experimentally impossible to prove or disprove the transmissibility of scrapie to man.

Lack of an inflammatory reaction, astrocytosis and spongy degeneration are not necessarily confined to spongiform encephalopathies caused by a slow virus infection. Similar lesions can be produced experimentally in infections with many acute viruses by subjecting the animals to immunosuppression (Zlotnik et al. 1970, 1971, 1972a). Thus it is possible to suggest the hypothesis that the agents of the spongiform encephalopathies exert an immunosuppressive effect on the host directed only against its own antigen and not against other antigens. This would explain the lack of antibody formation, absence of inflammatory reaction and spongiform degenerative changes. It has been shown that viruses may cause immunodepression, though in each case it is against another antigen not against its own. For example, measles virus tends to aggravate concurrent tuberculosis or malaria by causing immuno-depression against these agents (Smith 1970; Allison 1972).

PERSISTENT VIRAL INFECTIONS OF THE CENTRAL NERVOUS SYSTEM

A number of viral infections of the CNS may come under the above heading and they all differ from the previous group of slow virus infections in that there is persistence of virus in spite of the presence of immune responses, or that persistence of the viral infection was caused by an altered immunological response, such as immunodeficiency, or impaired immunological response to infection as in progressive multifocal leucoencephalopathy where papovavirus is reported to be implicated (Dayan 1969; Gajdusek 1972b). The term 'persistent viral infection' can be widely inter-preted. The persistence may be due to a prolongation of the incubation period, or to the actual illness, or to the continued presence of virus in the host whether giving rise to signs of disease or not (Waterson 1972). Some viruses like visna, a slow virus infection of sheep in Iceland, have a natural predilection for a slow persistent infection; other viruses that normally give rise to acute infections may, under conditions of altered host–virus relationship, cause a persistent infection, such as measles virus in subacute sclerosing panencephalitis (SSPE) or Russian spring–summer encephalitis virus in epilepsia partialis continua (Kojev-nikov) (Olitsky & Clarke 1959; Gajdusek 1972b).

Persistent viral infections without an impairment of the immunological response
Subacute sclerosing panencephalitis (SSPE) is the example for the naturally occurring persistent infections of the CNS giving rise to a subacute condition, although not necessarily degenerative, especially in the initial stages of the illness. The virus implicated in subacute sclerosing panencephalitis is measles virus. The virus

of SSPE is usually difficult to isolate from the brain of a patient, as it is cell-associated; however, once recovered by the method of co-culture it becomes almost indistinguishable from measles virus. Although differences have been reported between the SSPE agent and strains of measles virus, these are not sufficient to postulate a different virus and are compatible with differences due to variations in passage levels of the same virus (Horta-Barbosa et al. 1969, 1970; Ter Meulen et al. 1972).

SSPE occurs in children or in early adolescents and while very high levels of circulating antimeasles antibodies are invariably found, measles virus can also be demonstrated occasionally in brain biopsies. The disease usually runs a variable course and, in cases of short duration or early in the course of a protracted disease, apart from sclerotic changes and subacute inflammatory lesions, characteristic inclusion bodies can be found in the brain. In long-lasting or protracted cases with clinical histories of 5 to 9 years inflammation may be completely absent. In these instances there are usually Alzheimer's neurofibrillary changes in the neurones, demyelination of the white matter and severe astrocytosis in the grey matter (Plate VI/1). The intranuclear inclusions often demonstrated in the cerebral cortex in the early clinical periods, may be absent in the long standing cases (Herndon & Rubinstein 1968; Zeman & Kolar 1968). By using immunofluorescent techniques, the inclusion bodies give a positive reaction for measles virus. However when these inclusions are stained not with anti-measles labelled serum but with anti-human serum, the inclusions appear also stained, but in the form of diffuse fluorescence, suggesting that part of the inclusion body at least consists of globulins (Plate V/2, 3).

Several theories have been presented to explain the occurrence of SSPE in human patients. It has been suggested that SSPE is due to a failure of cellular immunity, thus preventing the eradication of intracellular measles antigen (Burnet 1968; Saunders et al. 1969; Gerson & Haslam 1971; Horta-Barbosa et al. 1971). Other authors put forward the hypothesis of dual infection by measles and papovavirus (Barbanti-Brodano et al. 1970; Brody & Detels 1970; Koprowski et al. 1970). There is no doubt, however, that whatever the cause of SSPE, the biological properties of the agent, isolated from brains of patients, show a great similarity to those of measles virus. At the same time, the agent has a convincing affinity for the CNS, either on direct transmission to ferrets (Katz et al. 1970) or after co-cultivation in a tissue culture system for hamsters (Byington et al. 1970; Byington & Johnson 1972).

The SSPE agent transmitted to baby hamsters and called the HBS virus (Byington & Johnson 1972) when inoculated into weanling hamsters gives rise to acute encephalitis, followed sometimes by a chronic disease. In such hamsters, infectious or cell-free virus was obtained during the first 8 days after inoculation. However, defective or cell-associated virus was demonstrated by co-cultivation methods for up till 81 days, while measles antigen was stained by immunofluorescent techniques for up to 55 days after infection. In animals affected by the chronic disease, subacute sclerotic lesions with cells containing eosinophilic nuclear inclusions persisted from 21 until 120 days after inoculation. Such weanling animals had also elevated HAI antibodies. Adult hamsters, however, inoculated with the HBS virus developed acute inflammatory lesions, which disappeared usually after 21 days. Virus was recovered from the brain of such animals only until the twelfth day after inoculation, while HAI (haemagglutination/inhibition) antibodies were demonstrated only until the thirtieth day.

A somewhat similar chronic encephalitis to that caused by the HBS virus was produced also in hamsters born to immunized mothers and infected with a hamster-adapted strain of measles virus (Wear & Rapp 1971). When such virus was inoculated into unprotected newborn hamsters there was acute encephalitis and death. However, if the mothers of the newborn hamsters were immunized against measles the infection remained latent until the infected hamsters were immunosuppressed with cyclophosphamide, when the majority developed a chronic disease with persistent myoclonic tremors. The explanation advanced was that humoral immunity acquired from the mothers blocked the cell associated infection in the brain, which became reactivated after immunosuppression. Although the above hypothesis appears to be

PLATE V

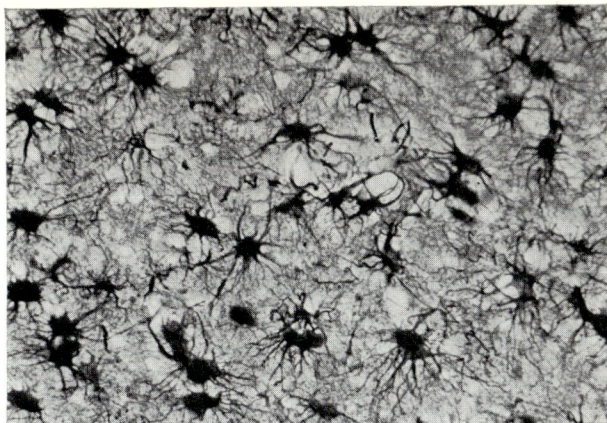

Fig. 1. Astrocytosis in the human cerebral cortex in Jakob–Creutzfeldt disease.

Cajal. × 200

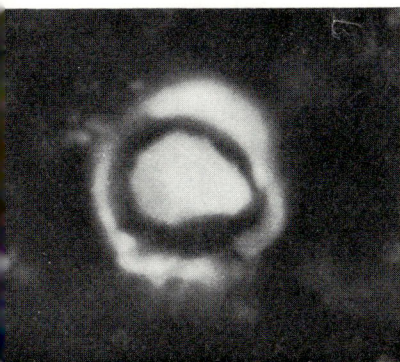

Fig. 2. Inclusion bodies in the human cerebral cortex in a patient suffering from subacute sclerosing panencephalitis, shown by means of immunofluorescence with anti-measles globulin.

Fluorescein isothiocyanate. × 1600

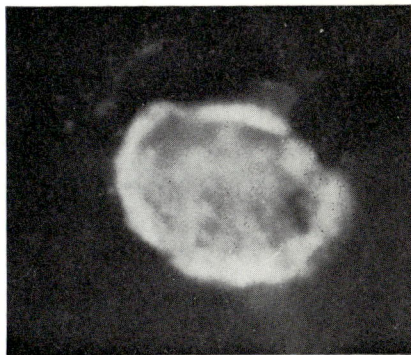

Fig. 3. Inclusion bodies in the human cerebral cortex of a patient suffering from subacute sclerosing panencephalitis, shown by means of immunofluorescence with anti-human globulin.

Fluorescein isothiocyanate. × 1600

PLATE VI

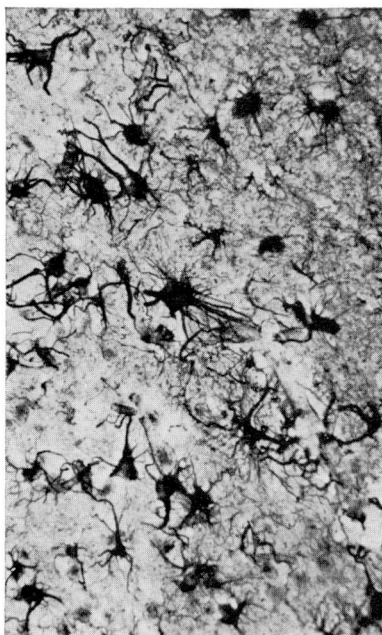

Fig. 1. Astrocytosis in the human cerebral cortex of a patient suffering from subacute sclerosing panencephalitis.

Cajal. × 200

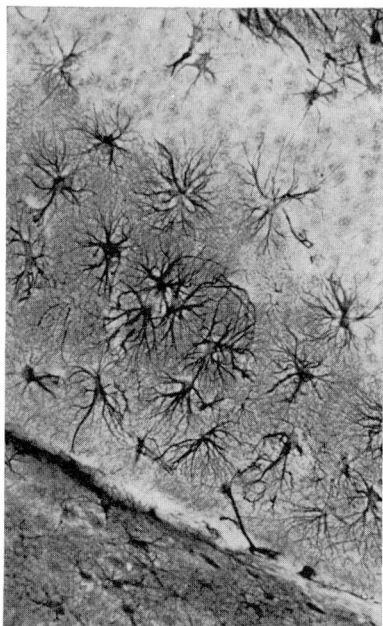

Fig. 2. Astrocytosis in the hippocampus of mice 26 months after inapparent infection with Semliki Forest Virus. Note the similarity to the lesion seen in mice affected with scrapie (Plate III/3).

Cajal. × 200

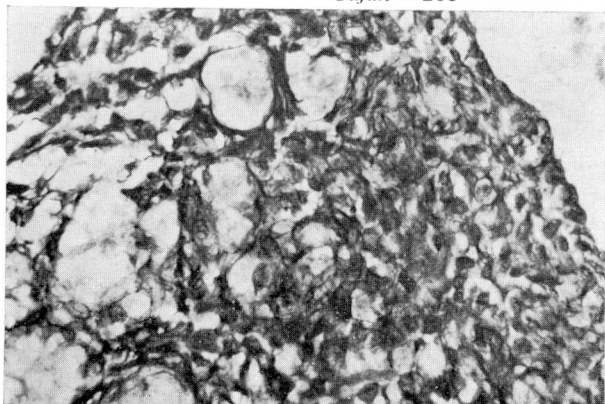

Fig. 3. Astrocytosis in the hippocampus of hamsters affected with subacute sclerosing encephalitis following infection with the HNT strain of measles virus.

Cajal. × 200

acceptable, the fact remains that another hamster-adapted strain of measles, the HNT strain (Burnstein et al. 1964; Burnstein & Byington 1968; Albrecht & Schumacher 1971) is capable of setting up a chronic CNS disease, not only in suckling or weanling hamsters, but also in adult hamsters. In a large study, the one hundred and forty-second hamster passage of the HNT strain of measles virus was used to infect adult hamsters by various routes. The results showed that hamsters of all ages were susceptible to the infection by almost all known routes of inoculation, including intraperitoneal, intracerebral, intranasal and respiratory. Depending on the age of the hamsters a proportion of the inoculated animals developed acute encephalitis, which curiously enough ran a biphasic course with mortality either between 10 and 11 days or 19 and 20 days after infection. No animals developed signs or mortality, between the twelfth and eighteenth day. Three weeks after infection a proportion of hamsters which did not go down during the acute phase developed a subacute condition which persisted for several months with severe progressive sclerosis and atrophy of selected parts of the brain. The distribution of the sclerotic lesions in the brain of affected hamsters was closely related to the route of infection. Thus, hamsters infected intracerebrally had the most prominent changes in the hippocampus (Plate VI/3), while those given virus intranasally had the lesions located in the olfactory lobes, pyriform and entorhinal cortex, and only to a lesser extent in the hippocampus. Finally, intraperitoneally inoculated hamsters had lesions in the hippocampus, the frontal cortex and the parietal cortex.

In a series of experiments, various monkeys, including rhesus, vervet, patas, squirrel and spider, were inoculated either with hamster-adapted measles virus (HNT) or with the hamster adapted SSPE agent (HBS) and the results compared. It appears that after only 19 passages in suckling hamsters, the SSPE agent became pathogenic for monkeys when inoculated intracerebrally and proved much more virulent than the hamster-adapted neurotropic strain of measles (HNT) after even 142 passages in suckling hamsters. When the HNT strain in its one hundred and sixteenth passage was inoculated intracerebrally into rhesus monkeys there was an inapparent infection with brain lesions 21 days after inoculation. However when such intracerebrally inoculated monkeys were treated with cyclophosphamide, 4 of 5 monkeys developed clinical signs 2 to $3\frac{1}{2}$ weeks later, leading to prostration and death (Albrecht & Schumacher 1971). Further passages of the HNT strain in suckling hamsters did not enhance its virulence for monkeys. The one hundred and forty-second passage of the HNT strain inoculated into patas monkeys did not give rise to clinical signs, but when monkeys were immunosuppressed 2 out of 4 patas monkeys developed clinical encephalitis and died 10 days later, one monkey became permanently paralysed and the last one remained in good health for 3 months after inoculation.

The HBS strain of SSPE agent, on the other hand, while showing almost no virulence for monkeys after 13 hamster passages, became decidedly virulent in the nineteenth passage and gave rise to clinical signs and mortality in intracerebral inoculated monkeys, irrespective of whether immunosuppressed or not between the tenth and twenty-fifth day after inoculation. Only 1 of 6 inoculated non-immunosuppressed monkeys did not die after the onset of clinical signs. This monkey remained ill and prostrated for 10 days and thereafter started showing signs of improvement. All non-immunosuppressed monkeys developing encephalitis had lesions throughout the brain and the spinal cord. Both degenerative and inflammatory changes were present and especially conspicuous were large granulomatous proliferations of astrocytes and microglia, often leading to the formation of small foci of malacia in the vicinity. The whole length of the spinal cord was invariably affected, the lesions being especially severe in the ventral horns. In the spinal cord of immunosuppressed monkeys no inflammation was present, but the ventral horn neurones were affected by chromatolysis and necrosis accompanied by neuronophagia. Similarly in the brain of immunosuppressed animals no inflammatory changes were seen. In the cerebellar folia degeneration of Purkinje cells was common and the molecular layer had marked microglial infiltrations. Foci of spongy degeneration were present in the medulla, pons, midbrain and thalamus. In the cerebral cortex swelling and degeneration of Betz cells was noticeable.

The tendency of a virus to change its pattern of infection from an acute to subacute or chronic is not necessarily confined to measles virus. Some attenuated strains of group A arboviruses (WEE and SFV) have the same predilection; similarly, a change of host from mouse to hamster had the same effect with Langat virus, a member of group B arboviruses. In each of the above subacute or chronic forms of encephalitis caused by arboviruses a persistent CNS infection was suspected although no evidence has yet been produced to prove it. Thus an attenuated vaccine strain of WEE (western equine encephalitis) virus, clone 15-variant, caused fatal encephalitis in suckling hamsters up to the age of 12 days old. However, 15-day-old hamsters, when inoculated with the virus either intracerebrally or peripherally, survived the infection. In the brains of these surviving hamsters the acute lesions of encephalitis slowly disappeared and were followed by subacute changes in the form of huge granulomatous cellular accumulations surrounded by spongy degeneration in various parts of the cerebral cortex (Zlotnik 1972a). The same clone of WEE, when inoculated into adult hamsters, produced a very mild encephalitis followed 14 days later by subacute sclerosis in the pyriform and entorhinal cortex. The subacute changes consisted of granulomatous microglial cell nests, very severe astrogliosis with the formation of long astrocytic processes arranged in dense tangles. This was followed by sclerotic changes, malacia, micro-cavitation and finally complete atrophy of affected parts (Zlotnik et al. 1972a).

Although the majority of strains of Semliki Forest virus (SFV) are virulent and lethal for adult mice, the A8 strain caused only an inapparent infection without clinical signs or mortality, but with the appearance of inflammatory brain lesions lasting for 3 to 6 weeks. When such recovered mice were allowed to live for over 2 years it was found that they developed a slow progressive encephalopathy leading to advanced hydrocephalus, spongy degeneration and marked astrocytic proliferation and hypertrophy in the cerebral cortex and in the hippocampus (Zlotnik et al. 1972b). Apart from the hydrocephalus, the lesions in the brain of the above mice resembled those of mice infected with scrapie (Plate VI/2).

Langat virus (TP21), closely related to other members of the tick-borne encephalitis group, is highly virulent for mice, but not for adult hamsters. An attenuated strain of Langat virus TP21-9 proved to be virulent and lethal only for newborn hamsters or those aged 1 to 3 days. Hamsters 5 days old developed an inapparent infection with inflammatory brain lesions, but without clinical signs (Zlotnik 1972a). However, about 35% of survivors after the disappearance of the initial changes of acute encephalitis developed a progressive subacute encephalitis with a very severe proliferation and hypertrophy of astrocytes, especially in the hippocampus, causing sclerosis and atrophy of the affected parts. A large proportion of survivors died during the 12 months following infection. In the brains of such mice there were noticeable subacute or chronic lesions and especially atrophy of the hippocampus. The virulent strain of TP21 proved to be lethal for suckling hamsters aged 1 to 12 days; 15-day-old hamsters inoculated with the virus developed a condition similar to that in 5-day-old hamsters inoculated with the attenuated clone TP21-9 (Zlotnik et al. 1973). Adult hamsters, on the other hand, proved to be resistant to both attenuated and virulent virus even when inoculated intracerebrally. When TP21 virus was passaged twice in newborn hamsters it became highly virulent for adult hamsters, but only when inoculated intracerebrally. About 40% of infected hamsters died from the disease during the first 3 weeks after inoculation. The course of the disease in hamsters was similar to that after HNT infection, being biphasic in character. Similarly about 70% of recovered hamsters developed subacute sclerotic changes accompanied by a very severe astrocytosis and atrophy of the hippocampus. The virulence of the virus was greatly enhanced after a further 17 passages in suckling hamsters, so that the nineteenth passage of TP21 caused a 100% mortality of adult hamsters after intracerebral inoculation. When given by intranasal instillations the virus gave rise to acute clinical encephalitis with mortality and a biphasic course of the disease in 40% of hamsters, while 50 to 60% of survivors developed subacute sclerosing lesions localized primarily in the olfactory lobes, pyriform cortex, entorhinal cortex and occasionally also the hippocampus.

Persistent infections in immunodeficient or immunosuppressed hosts

The effects of immunosuppression on viral encephalitis can be studied readily in experimental animals and the results obtained may prove of considerable value in understanding the problems involved in natural viral infections of patients affected with many forms of immunodeficiency disease (Dayan 1971). In viral infections of the CNS in immunodeficient hosts, irrespective of whether natural or experimental, there is usually suppression or complete absence of an inflammatory reaction in the brain and spinal cord and an upsurge of degenerative change accompanied by an astrogliosis. The above brain lesions appear to be very similar to changes characteristic of the spongiform encephalopathies caused by slow virus infection.

Immunosuppression not only makes the host more susceptible to viral infection but, by inhibiting the immune mechanism of the host, creates conditions suitable for the persistance of virus in the CNS and gives rise to increased viral replication to levels much higher than those ever obtained in non-immunosuppressed hosts (Nathanson & Cole 1970; Zlotnik et al. 1970, 1971). In experimental louping ill of guinea pigs for example the highest levels of virus in the CNS were estimated to be $10^{2.5}$ MLD_{50}/g, while in immunosuppressed animals levels of $10^{4.8}$ MLD_{50}/g were obtained.

Viral complications may follow not only various forms of immunodeficiency disease, but also other chronic conditions that cause an impaired immunological response to infection. It is thought that progressive multifocal leucoencephalopathy is caused by papovavirus infection as a complication to diseases such as Hodgkin's disease, chronic leukaemias, carcinomatosis and miliary tuberculosis. In addition to such complications, lesions characteristic of virus infection in immunodeficient hosts may be obtained experimentally in animals such as monkeys infected peripherally with the virus of WEE, where there was no penetration of the CNS by the virus. There was, however, a viraemia with subsequent formation of antibodies. Intranasal or intracerebral challenge of these monkeys gave rise to signs of acute encephalitis in some of the animals. The brains of the above monkeys had very severe degenerative lesions and astrogliosis, but no inflammatory changes (Zlotnik et al. 1970). A similar effect was obtained in mice immunized peripherally against the virus of louping ill and then challenged by the intracerebral route. The explanation of the above phenomena is that the initial infection did not prime the brain and therefore a direct second infection of the CNS found the central nervous tissue susceptible to the virus, without, however, the possibility of recourse to the peripheral immune defences. Thus degenerative forms of encephalitis resembling natural degenerative conditions may occur when the immune responses of the host are either absent, abolished or altered.

SEQUELAE TO ACUTE VIRUS INFECTIONS

After the cessation of the acute phase, many viral infections of the CNS have the tendency to leave focal, subacute or chronic lesions, which may cause brain damage accompanied by signs such as intellectual deterioration, convulsions, muscular weakness and paralysis. Children are especially prone to permanent sequelae after encephalitis (Zlotnik 1972a). Of the viral infections that show the greatest tendency for sequelae that cause mental changes, the best known are those caused by arboviruses, especially of group A (WEE and EEE).

Western equine encephalitis (WEE) sometimes gives rise to the formation of permanent changes, mainly in children, in the form of focal CNS degeneration, cavitation and calcification (Davis 1940; Noran & Baker 1945). Eastern equine encephalitis (EEE) is a more serious condition than the preceding and, apart from causing great mortality, many recovered patients including adults develop very serious sequelae. These may vary from emotional instability to various types of paralysis and mental deterioration, usually accompanied by destruction of neurones in the CNS, malacia and spongy degeneration (Olitsky & Casals 1959). In group B arboviruses, sequelae are less common, but they do occur in diseases such as Japanese B encephalitis, and St Louis encephalitis, Russian spring–summer encephalitis and occasionally West Nile fever (Olitsky & Clarke 1959; Nisenbaum & Wallis 1965).

DISEASES OF THE CENTRAL NERVOUS SYSTEM OF POSSIBLE VIRAL AETIOLOGY

Of the various degenerative conditions of the CNS where a viral aetiology could be postulated, the following have attracted the greatest attention: disseminated sclerosis, amyotropical lateral sclerosis, Parkinson's disease and amyotropical lateral sclerosis–Parkinsonism dementia complex on Guam (Cathala & Brown 1972; Gibbs & Gadjusek 1972). There does not seem to be any doubt that there is a wealth of evidence supporting the theory of an infectious origin of these diseases however, though the infective agents have still not been demonstrated.

SUMMARY

A review of the many forms of virus infection of the CNS tends to point to a common pattern between acute, subacute, persistent and slow virus infections. This view is especially strengthened by the fact that many acute infections, under altered host–virus relations, may give rise to subacute degenerative conditions. Finally, the appearance of brain lesions in acute viral infections of immunosuppressed animals, resembling those of slow virus infections of the spongiform encephalopathy type, suggests a link between encephalitis in immunodeficient hosts and slow virus infections where no immune reactions were demonstrated.

REFERENCES

Allison, A. C. (1972) Immune responses in persistent virus infections. *J. clin. Path.*, **25**, Suppl. 6, 121.

Albrecht, P. & Schumacher, H. P. (1971) Neutrotropic properties of measles virus in hamsters and mice. *J. infect. Dis.*, **124**, 86.

Albrecht, P., Shibo, A. L., Burns, G. R. & Tauraso, N. M. (1972) Experimental measles encephalitis in normal and cyclophosphamide treated rhesus monkeys. *J. infect. Dis.*, **126**, 154.

Alper, T. (1972) The nature of the scrapie agent. *J. clin. Path.*, **25**, Suppl. 6, 154.

Barbanti-Brodano, G., Oyanagi, S., Katz, M., Koprowski, H. (1970) Presence of two different viral agents in cells of patients with sub-acute sclerosing panencephalitis. *Proc. Soc. exp. Biol. Med.*, **134**, 230.

Barlow, R. M. (1972) Transmissible mink encephalopathy: pathogenesis and nature of the etiological agent. *J. clin. Path.*, **25**, Suppl. 6, 102.

Brody, J. A. (1972) Epidemiologic and serologic data on multiple sclerosis and their possible significance in multiple sclerosis. *UCLA Forum in Medical Sciences*, No. 16, ed. Wolfgram, F., Ellison, G., Stevens, J., & Andrews, J., pp. 127–40. New York: Academic Press.

Brody, J. A. & Detels, R. (1970) Subacute sclerosing panencephalitis: A zoonosis following aberrant measles. *Lancet*, **ii**, 500.

Brody, J. A., Detels, R. & Sever, J. L. (1972) Measles—antibody titres in sibships of patients with subacute sclerosing panencephalitis and controls. *Lancet*, **i**, 177.

Brotherston, J. G., Renwick, C. C., Stamp, J. T., Zlotnik, I. & Pattison, I. H. (1968) Spread of scrapie by contact to goats and sheep. *J. comp. Path.*, **78**, 9.

Burnet, F. M. (1968) Measles as an index for immunological function. *Lancet*, **ii**, 610.

Burnstein, T. & Byington, D. P. (1968) On the isolation of measles virus from infected brain tissue: experimental measles encephalitis in the baby rat. *Neurology, Minneap.*, **18**, 162.

Burnstein, T., Jensen, J. H. & Waksman, B. H. (1964) The development of a neurotropic strain of measles virus in hamsters and mice. *J. infect. Dis.*, **114**, 265.

Byington, D. P., Castro, A. E. & Burnstein, T. (1970) Adaptation to hamsters of neurotropic measles virus from subacute sclerosing panencephalitis. *Nature, Lond.*, **225**, 554.

Byington, D. P. & Johnson, K. P. (1972) Experimental SSPE in the hamster: correlation of age with chronic inclusion cell encephalitis. *J. infect. Dis.*, **126**, 18.

Cathala, F. & Brown, P. (1972) The possible viral etiology of disseminated sclerosis. *J. clin. Path.*, **25**, Suppl. 6, 141.

Chandler, R. L. (1961) Encephalopathy in mice produced by inoculation with scrapie brain material. *Lancet*, **i**, 1378.

Chandler, R. L. & Fisher, J. (1963) Experimental transmission of scrapie to rats. *Lancet*, **ii**, 1165.

Daniel, P. M. (1971) Transmissible degenerative diseases of the nervous system. *Proc. R. soc. Med.*, **64**, 787.

Daniel, P. M. (1972) Creutzfeldt-Jakob Disease. *J. clin. Path.*, **25**, Suppl. 6, 97.

Davis, J. H. (1940) Equine encephalomyelitis (western type) in children. *J. Pediat.*, **16**, 591.

Dayan, A. D. (1969) Progressive multifocal leukoencephalopathy. In *Virus Diseases and the Nervous System*, ed. Whitty, C. W. M., Hughes, J. T. & MacCallum, F. O., pp. 199–206. Oxford: Blackwell Scientific.

Dayan, A. D. (1971) Chronic encephalitis in children with severe immuno deficiency. *Acta neuropath.*, **19**, 234.

Dickinson, A. G., Mackay, J. M. K. & Zlotnik, I. (1964) Transmission by contact of scrapie in mice. *J. comp. Path.*, **74**, 250.

Field, E. J. (1968) Transmission of kuru to mice. *Lancet*, **i**, 981.

Field, E. J. (1969) Slow virus infections of the nervous system. *Int. Rev. exp. Path.*, **8**, 130.

Gajdusek, D. C. (1972a) Slow infections: spongiform virus encephalopathies. *J. clin. Path.*, **25**, Suppl. 6, 78.

Gajdusek, D. C. (1972b) Slow virus infection and activation of latent infections in ageing. *Adv. Gerontol. Res.*, **4**, 201.

Gerson, K. L. & Haslam, R. H. A. (1971) Subtle immunologic abnormalities in four boys with subacute sclerosing panencephalitis. *New Engl. J. Med.*, **285**, 78.

Gibbs, C. J., jun. & Gajdusek, D. C. (1972a) Isolation and characterisation of the subacute spongiform virus encephalopathies of man: Kuru and Creutzfeldt–Jakob disease. *J. clin. Path.*, **25**, Suppl. 6, 84.

Gibbs, C. J., jun. & Gajdusek, D. C. (1972b) Amytrophic lateral sclerosis, Parkinson's disease and the amyotrophic lateral sclerosis–Parkinsonism–dementia complex of Guam: A review and summary of attempts to demonstrate infection as the etiology. *J. clin. Path.*, **25**, Suppl. 6, 132.

Gibbs, C. J., jun. & Gajdusek, D. C. (1972c) Transmission of scrapie to the cynomolgus monkey (*Macaca fascicularis*). *Nature, Lond.*, **236**, 73.

Herndon, R. M. & Rubinstein, L. J. (1968) Light and electron microscopy observations on the development of viral particles in the inclusions of Dawson's encephalitis (subacute sclerosing panencephalitis). *Neurology, Minneap.*, **18**, 8.

Horta-Barbosa, L., Fucillo, D. A., Hamilton, R., Traub, R., Ley, A. & Sever, J. L. (1970) Some characteristics of SSPE measles virus. *Proc. Soc. exp. Biol.*, **134**, 17.

Horta-Barbosa, L., Fucillo, D. A., London, W. T., Jabbour, J. Z., Zeman, W. & Sever, J. L. (1969) Isolation of measles virus from brain cell cultures of two patients with subacute sclerosing panencephalitis. *Proc. Soc. exp. Biol.*, **132**, 272.

Horta-Barbosa, L., Hamilton, R., Witting, B., Fucillo, D. A., Sever,

J. L. & Vernon, M. (1971) Subacute sclerosing panencephalitis: isolation of suppressed measles virus from lymph node biopses. *Science, N.Y.*, **173**, 840.

Katz, M., Rorke, L. B., Masland, W. S., Barbanti-Brodano, G. & Koprowski, H. (1970) Subacute sclerosing panencephalitis: isolation of a virus encephalitogenic for ferrets. *J. infect. Dis.*, **121**, 188.

Koprowski, H., Barbanti-Brodano, G. & Katz, M. (1970) Interaction between papova-like virus and paramyxovirus in human brain cells. A hypothesis. *Nature, Lond.*, **225**, 1045.

Lampert, P. W., Gajdusek, D. C. & Gibbs, C. J., jun. (1972) Subacute spongiform virus encephalopathies. Scrapie, kuru and Creutzfeldt-Jakob disease: A review. *Am. J. Path.*, **68**, 626.

Marsh, R. F., Burger, D., Eckroade, R., Zu Rhein, G. M. & Hanson, R. P. (1969a) A preliminary report on the experimental host range of the transmissible mink encephalopathy agent. *J. infect. Dis.*, **120**, 713.

Marsh, R. F., Burger, D. & Hanson, R. P. (1969b) Transmissible mink encephalopathy: behaviour of the disease agent in mink. *Am. J. vet. Res.*, **30**, 1637.

Marsh, R. F. & Hanson, R. P. (1969) Physical and chemical properties of the transmissible mink encephalopathy agent. *J. Virol.*, **3**, 176.

Nathanson, N. & Cole, G. A. (1970) Fatal Japanese encephalitis virus infection in immunosuppressed spider monkeys. *Clin. exp. Immunol.* **6**, 161.

Nisenbaum, C. & Wallis, K. (1965) Meningo-encephalitis due to West Nile fever. *Helv. paediat. Acta*, **20**, 392.

Noran, H. H. & Baker, A. B. (1945) Western equine encephalitis: The pathogenesis of the pathological lesions. *J. Neuropath. exp. Neurol.*, **4**, 269.

Olitsky, P. K. & Casals, J. (1959) Arthropod-borne Group A virus infections of man. In *Viral and Rickettsial Infections of Man*, ed. Rivers, T. M. and Horsfall, F. L. London: Pitman Medical.

Olitsky, P. K. & Clarke, D. H. (1959) Arthropod-borne Group B virus infections of man. In *Viral and Rickettsial Infections of Man*, ed. Rivers, T. M. & Horsfall, F. L. London: Pitman Medical.

Pattison, I. H. (1965) Resistance of the scrapie agent to formalin. *J. comp. Path.*, **75**, 159.

Porter, D. D. (1972) Mechanisms of slow virus infection and possible relevance to multiple sclerosis. In *Multiple Sclerosis UCLA Forum in Medical Sciences, No. 16*, ed. Wolfgram, F., Ellison, G., Stevens, J. & Andrews, J., pp. 233–43. New York : Academic Press.

Saunders, M., Knowles, M., Chamber, M. E., Caspary, E. A., Gardner-Medwin, D. & Walker, P. (1969) Cellular and humoral responses to measles in subacute sclerosing panencephalitis. *Lancet*, **i**, 72.

Smith, G. C. E. (1970) Immunology and virus diseases. *J. R. Coll. Phycns., Lond.*, **5**, 31.

Stamp, J. T., Brotherston, J. G., Zlotnik, I. Mackay, J. M. K. & Smith, W. (1959) Further studies on scrapie. *J. comp. Path.*, **69**, 268.

Ter Meulen, V., Katz, M., Kackel, Y. M., Barbanti-Brodano, G. & Koprowski, H. (1972) Subacute sclerosing panencephalitis. *In vitro* characterization of viruses isolated from brain cells in culture. *J. infect. Dis.*, **126**, 11.

Waterson, A. P. (1972) Host–virus relationship with special reference to Newcastle disease and serum hepatitis. *J. clin. Path.*, **25**, Suppl. 6, 1.

Wear, D. J. & Rapp, F. (1971) Latent measles virus infection of the hamster central nervous system. *J. Immunol.*, **107**, 1543.

Zeman, W. & Kolar, O. (1968) Reflections on the etiology and pathogenesis of subacute sclerosing panencephalitis. *Neurology, Minneap.*, **18**, 1.

Zlotnik, I. (1958a) The histopathology of the brain stem of sheep affected with natural scrapie. *J. comp. Path.*, **68**, 411.

Zlotnik, I. (1958b) The histopathology of the brain stem of sheep affected with experimental scrapie. *J. comp. Path.*, **68**, 428.

Zlotnik, I. (1961) The histopathology of the brain of goats affected with scrapie. *J. comp. Path.*, **71**, 440.

Zlotnik, I. (1962a) The pathology of scrapie: A comparative study of lesions in the brain of sheep and goats. *Acta neuropath.*, Suppl. 1, 61.

Zlotnik, I. (1962b) A comparative study of early lesions in the brain of goats inoculated with scrapie goat brain by the intracerebral and the subcutaneous routes. *J. comp. Path.*, **72**, 366.

Zlotnik, I. (1963) Experimental transmission of scrapie to golden hamsters. *Lancet*, **ii**, 1072.

Zlotnik, I. (1965) Observations on the experimental transmission of scrapie of various origins to laboratory animals. In *Slow, Latent and Temperate Viruses*, ed. Gadjuseh, D. C., Gibbs, J. C. & Alpers, M., p. 237. NINDB Monograph No. 2, U.S. Department of Health, Education and Welfare.

Zlotnik, I. (1968a) Spread of scrapie by contact in mice. *J. comp. Path.*, **78**, 19.

Zlotnik, I. (1968b) The reaction of astrocytes to acute virus infections of the central nervous system. *Br. J. exp. Path.*, **49**, 555.

Zlotnik, I. (1970) The pathogenesis of scrapie. *Proc. VIth int. Congr. Neuropath.*, 901.

Zlotnik, I. (1972a) Virus infection and brain development in brain in unclassified mental retardation study Group No. 3—Institute for Research into Mental Retardation, ed. Cavanagh, J. B., Edinburgh and London: Churchill Livingstone.

Zlotnik, I. (1972b) The role of immune reactions in viral encephalitis. *Proc. 3rd int. Congr. Neuro-Genetics and Neuro-Ophthal., Brussels*, **6**, 185.

Zlotnik, I. & Barlow, R. M. (1967) The transmission of a specific encephalopathy of mink to the goat. *Vet. Rec.*, **81**, 55.

Zlotnik, I., Carter, G. B. & Grant, D. P. (1971) The persistence of louping-ill virus in immunosuppressed guinea pigs. *Br. J. exp. Path.*, **52**, 395.

Transmissible and degenerative diseases

Zlotnik, I. & Grant, D. P. (1973) The relationship between immunity and the pathology of the CNS of mice infected with CVS strain of rabies. *Br. J. exp. Path.*, **54**, 534.

Zlotnik, I., Grant, D. P. & Batter-Hatton, D. (1972b) Encephalopathy in mice following inapparent Semliki Forest virus (SFV) infection. *Br. J. exp. Path.*, **53**, 125.

Zlotnik, I., Grant, D. P., Carter, G. B. & Batter-Hatton, D. (1973) Subacute sclerosing encephalitis in adult hamsters infected with langat virus. *Br. J. exp. Path.*, **54**, 29.

Zlotnik, I., Peacock, S., Grant, D. P. & Batter-Hatton, D. (1972a) The pathogenesis of western equine encephalitis virus (WEE) in adult hamsters with special reference to the long- and short-term effects on the CNS of the attenuated clone 15 variant. *Br. J. exp. Path.*, **53**, 59.

Zlotnik, I. & Rennie, J. C. (1962) The pathology of the brain of mice inoculated with tissues from scrapie sheep. *J. comp. Path.*, **72**, 360.

Zlotnik, I. & Rennie, J. C. (1963) Further observations on the experimental transmission of scrapie from sheep and goats to laboratory mice. *J. comp. Path.*, **73**, 150.

Zlotnik, I. & Rennie, J. C. (1965) Experimental transmission of mouse passaged scrapie to goats, sheep, rats and hamsters. *J. comp. Path.*, **75**, 147.

Zlotnik, I. & Rennie, J. C. (1967) The effect of heat on the scrapie agent in mouse brain. *Br. J. exp. Path.*, **48**, 171.

Zlotnik, I., Smith, C. E. G., Grant, D. P. & Peacock, S. (1970) The effect of immunosuppression on viral encephalitis with special reference to cyclophosphamide. *Br. J. exp. Path.*, **51**, 434.

Zlotnik, I. & Stamp, J. T. (1965) Scrapie in a Dorset Down ram. A confirmation of the histological diagnosis by means of intracerebral inoculation of mice with formol fixed brain tissue. *Vet. Rec.*, **77**, 1178.

Zlotnik, I. & Stamp, J. T. (1966) The transmission of scrapie from a Dorset Down ram to Cheviot sheep by means of intracerebral inoculations of formol fixed brain tissue. *Vet. Rec.*, **78**, 222.

9

The Clinical Aspects of Slow Virus Infections of the Human Brain

W. B. MATTHEWS

When Jakob–Creutzfeldt disease was regarded as merely one of a number of infinitely depressing degenerative diseases of the nervous system causing pre-senile dementia, and kuru was thought to be a hereditary cerebellar degeneration confined to a single exotic tribe, the clinical features of these diseases were naturally of little general interest, even to neurologists. Controversy on the identity of Jakob–Creutzfeldt disease (JCD) certainly existed almost from the first descriptions by von Economo and Schilder (1920), Creutzfeldt (1920) and Jakob (1921a, b) and was accentuated by the description of an apparently related condition by Jones and Nevin (1954) and by Nevin et al. (1960). Many classifications were proposed (Kirschbaum 1968; van Rossum 1968), usually based on an uneasy combination of clinical and pathological findings, but their lack of precision is illustrated by the invariable need for transitional types or subdivisions. The main discussion has recently centred on whether two diseases exist: the spastic pseudosclerosis of Jakob and the spongiform encephalopathy of Jones and Nevin (Nevin et al. 1967). These titles, admittedly rather selected, emphasize the difficulties of contrasting one group, defined largely on clinical features, with another in which pathology is the main criterion. Other less substantial dividing lines were drawn between groups with differing presenting symptoms or distribution of lesions at autopsy. The perhaps rather slender interest of this elaborate and necessarily inconclusive debate was abruptly enhanced by the discovery that at least one form was transmissible to primates (Gibbs et al. 1968) in a manner comparable to the laboratory transmission of kuru (Gajdusek et al. 1966) and under conditions qualifying for the title of 'slow virus infection'. Discussion can now be more sharply focussed on specific aspects. For example, are all forms of the disease transmissible in the laboratory? Are kuru and JCD perhaps caused by the same agent modified by differing hosts? Is JCD naturally transmissible? As laboratory experiments on slow viruses are by definition extremely protracted the clinical evidence must also be scrutinized for additional information.

CLINICAL IDENTIFICATION OF JCD

I have attempted to review the clinical and epidemiological features of patients diagnosed at autopsy or biopsy as having JCD, subacute spongiform encephalopathy or corticostriatospinal atrophy in England and Wales. For many reasons there can be no possibility of a complete survey and in general information has been obtained on patients diagnosed since 1966, with some earlier cases from selected centres. This study is still in progress and only partial results on 49 patients can be reported.

Age of onset and duration
The duration of the disease, at least as far as overt symptomatology is concerned, can usually be established with some certainty. It is true that on close questioning of relatives a history of minor symptoms long preceding the onset of severe disease may occasionally be obtained, but in the 12 patients in whom I have personally conducted such enquiry, trivial and fluctuating disturbances of mood of doubtful relevance had been noted only in 2. Of 46 patients in whom the interval between the onset of recognizable symptoms and death is known the duration of the disease was 12 months or less in all but 9 (Fig. 6). In the remaining 9 the duration

was from 20 months to $4\frac{3}{4}$ years. (The duration was not known in 3 patients. One is still alive but clearly falls into the long survival group. In 2 the precise date of death has not yet been ascertained but both were moribund within 6 months of the onset.) The

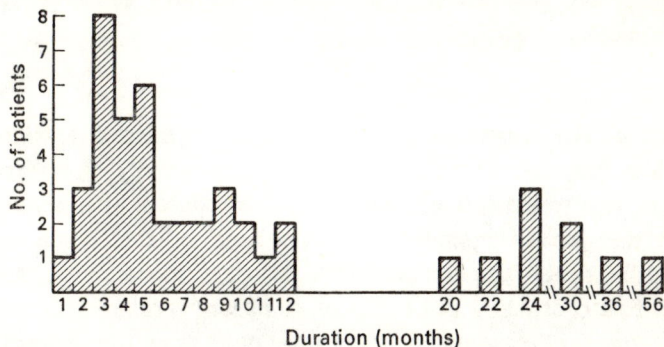

Fig. 6. The duration of Jakob–Creutzfeldt disease in patients in whom this could be clearly established.

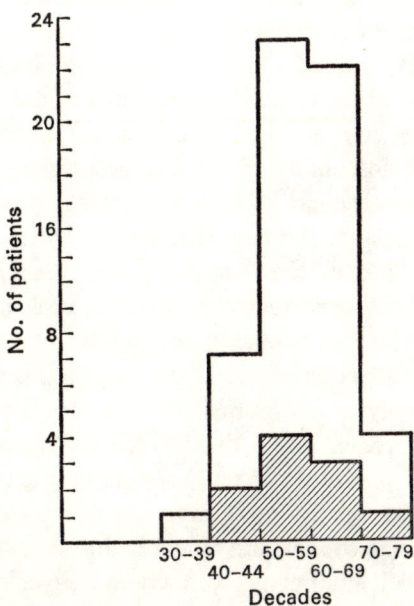

Fig. 7. Age of onset of Jakob–Creutzfeldt disease; the shaded area indicates those patients with disease of long duration.

numbers are too small to be certain that with regard to duration there is a bimodal pattern, and other collected series have shown a steady fall from a peak duration of around 6 to 9 months (van Rossum 1968). The age at onset did not differ in these two groups (Fig. 7) but analysis of other clinical features shows further differences.

Clinical picture

Many of the larger group of 39 patients presented a clinical picture unmistakably that of a subacute rapidly progressive disease that would scarcely call to mind the concept of a 'degenerative' disorder. One patient, indeed, became bed-ridden one week from the onset of the first symptom. Although the initial diagnosis was often considered to be that of an acute psychiatric disorder, thereafter the differential diagnosis was more often from encephalitis or brain tumour. In a rapidly progressive dementing disease the identification of the presenting symptom is naturally inexact, but in 17 patients disturbance of higher cerebral functions had originally suggested a primary psychiatric disease. The relatively abrupt onset of lack of interest, depression, inability to concentrate, failing memory and confusion in a middle-aged patient, without apparent relation to focal cerebral dysfunction, inevitably leads to the diagnosis of an affective disorder. One patient in the fourth decade was thought to have schizophrenia and one patient with cortical blindness and one with dizziness were considered to have hysteria. The precise nature of the disability was often difficult to establish, particularly as this phase was usually rapidly overtaken by the development of unmistakable evidence of organic disease affecting cortical or subcortical structures. The retrospective analysis of 'confusion' from the impressions of a distraught relative, or from the incoherent mutterings of the patient, seldom permitted any precise localization of the initial cerebral disturbance. Forgetfulness, dysphasia, disorientation, inability to localize sounds and visual hallucinations could all be recognized in individual patients in whom a psychiatric diagnosis was at first considered probable.

In 10 patients the initial complaint was of dizziness or of

definite rotatory vertigo. Here again the rapid appearance of other symptoms leading to obviously important disability prevented any diagnostic confusion with banal causes of dizziness. Five patients initially complained of an unsteady gait and it is probable that in a number of patients a complaint of dizziness implied ataxia. Visual symptoms in various combinations of cortical blindness and hallucinations were the presenting feature in 5 patients. In 2 patients weakness of one limb was the first complaint; one patient presented with obvious dysphasia and one with diplopia. Two patients appear twice in this list of presenting symptoms because focal signs were misinterpreted as due to psychiatric disease.

In this group of patients the subsequent clinical course was decline within a few weeks or months into a state of increasing helplessness. The stages by which this was reached varied greatly in detail from one patient to another. Failure of intellectual functions proceeded rapidly and severe dementia was an invariable feature. Speech became severely disturbed, most patients eventually becoming mute. Detailed analysis of the speech disorder was not practicable in the presence of disorientation and memory failure, but initially the defect was often recognizable as dysphasic, usually with severe defects of comprehension. At a later stage, when swallowing had also become disturbed, speech mechanisms were obviously involved at a bulbar or pseudobulbar level. Some evidence of cortical blindness was detected in 11 patients and may, of course, have affected others who could not be adequately tested. Terrifying visual hallucinations formed a prominent but mercifully brief episode in one of my own patients. Auditory hallucinations were not reported.

Signs of cerebellar dysfunction, mainly affecting the gait, were prominent in 14 patients but did not persist for long in isolation. Increase in tone in the limbs, variously described as spasticity or rigidity but usually the latter, was a universal feature but seldom occurred early in the course of the disease. Eventually a state of decerebrate or decorticate rigidity supervened in many patients, but others died in coma without having adopted these stereotyped postures. Fluctuating rigidity was often noted but cog-wheel rigidity was not recorded. The plantar reflexes were often difficult to evaluate and precise figures would not be meaningful, but extensor responses were common. On the other hand, a patient might be severely incapacitated at a stage when the plantars were clearly flexor. Increase in tendon reflexes was often reported in the early stages of the disease. Sensory functions were naturally often difficult or impossible to test but in the early stages sensory loss of cortical type was reported in 2 patients. The cause of the diplopia in the patient who presented with this symptom was not determined.

Severe muscular wasting of the degree found in motor neurone disease was not encountered in this group of patients. Some evidence of anterior horn cell involvement was suspected in 2 patients but terminal cachexia was naturally common and in patients personally observed the degree of wasting did not obviously exceed that expected in an inert patient.

Involuntary movements were common, that most frequently encountered being myoclonus, which was recorded in 35 of these patients. The myoclonus of JCD is often preceded by other forms of involuntary movement, in particular a widespread or generalized startle reaction in response to noise. Athetosis was recorded in 2 patients and one patient of my own had asterixis before myoclonus developed. When fully established the myoclonus is a sudden localized contraction often at a high rate of repetition at one site, for example one side of the face, then switching to an unrelated area. It usually reaches maximum intensity about the time the patient adopts the flexed decorticate posture and thereafter declines and eventually stops. Epileptic fits, either generalized or focal motor seizures, occurred in 7 patients but not in the early stages of the disease and serial fits presented a therapeutic problem only in one patient.

In the group of 10 patients in whom the disease ran a prolonged course the initial symptoms differed in some respects. Six patients were demented for a period of several months before other evidence of organic disease was observed. One patient presented with tremor, apparently not of parkinsonian type, two had weakness of one limb and one was initially dysarthric. Apart from the relatively slow development of the disease there were other notable differences from the first group of patients. In 6 of these 10 patients wasting was widespread and unmistakably due to anterior horn cell disease and not to cachexia. For example, in my own patient in this group examination at the stage when dementia was the only complaint revealed fasciculation in all muscles of the upper limbs and shoulder girdle. In contrast, only 2 of these patients developed myoclonus, in none was visual loss recorded and clinical evidence of cerebellar dysfunction was not prominent.

The clinical features of the first and much the larger group in general resemble those attributed to subacute spongiform encephalopathy (Nevin et al. 1960) and the differing emphasis on certain symptoms in the initial stages does not seem adequate grounds for further subdivision. It must be remembered that pathological changes cannot always be reflected in clinical signs. A patient who, I was told, from a pathological point of view 'must have been ataxic' from severe cerebellar disease had been incapable of any voluntary movement, ataxic or otherwise, for 3 months before he died. The validity of differentiating a Heidenhain's visual type (Heidenhain 1929) or an ataxic form (Brownell & Oppenheimer 1965) is difficult to maintain when the overlap of both clinical and pathological features is so extensive.

In the group of patients in whom the disease was of longer duration 6 conformed to an amyotrophic type in which a relatively protracted course is well recognized (van Rossum 1968). It is not possible, however, to equate the remaining 4 patients in this group with the spastic pseudosclerosis of Jakob. Nevin et al. (1967) have emphasized that Jakob's patients had early and prominent mental symptoms and signs of pyramidal and extra-pyramidal disease and apparently did not enter a terminal state of decerebrate or decorticate rigidity. The duration of the disease in the patients Jakob described is difficult to evaluate, partly because they were afflicted with other diseases that he was able to recognize as irrelevant. Probably the range is from 6 to 15 months (average 10 months) which is longer than the mean of 5·6 months of the more acute form in the present series but much shorter than that of any patient in the more chronic group. It must not be overlooked that in a number of respects Jakob's patients had symptoms commonly encountered in the more acute group in the present series. Thus, all 5 of Jakob's patients had involuntary movements, some apparently myoclonic, and 3 were ataxic. The decerebrate state was not described but in the present series a number of patients in both groups died in coma with intercurrent infection without reaching this state. Before the advent of modern nursing techniques and antibiotics such an eventuality would surely have been much more probable. I do not believe that a sharp distinction can be drawn on purely clinical grounds between the subacute spongiform encephalopathy of Jones and Nevin and the spastic pseudosclerosis of Jakob.

A more important distinction would be between a transmissible and a non-transmissible form of the disease as this would imply a real aetiological difference. The patients in the first more acute group in the present series approximate very closely to the clinical features of transmissible JCD described by Roos et al. (1973) and indeed 3 of the patients appear in both series. It is at present impossible to tell whether Gibbs and Gajdusek's group have identified a non-transmissible form because the incubation period of this type of agent may be extremely long, as shown by the $5\frac{1}{2}$-year incubation in transmission of scrapie to the monkey (Gibbs & Gajdusek 1972) and $8\frac{1}{2}$ years for transmission of kuru to the rhesus monkey (Gajdusek & Gibbs 1972). However Roos et al. (1973) comment that in the group of patients from whom transmission had not yet been successful there was a higher incidence of prolonged duration and of prominent lower motor neurone signs and a relative infrequency of myoclonus, features resembling those of the more chronic group identified in the present series. The patient S. F., stated in a footnote to Roos et al.'s paper to have had transmissible disease, is included in the present series and might well satisfy Nevin et al.'s (1967) criteria for Jakob's disease as she had prominent mental symptoms, with evidence of pyramidal and extrapyramidal disease, no myoclonus and no terminal decerebrate posture.

Differential diagnosis

The clinical features of the different stages of JCD clearly overlap with those of many other diseases of the nervous system. Mistaken diagnosis of a primary psychiatric disorder is unavoidable in the early stages of the disease in many patients. It should, however, be possible to suspect the presence of organic disease before the appearance of such unmistakable evidence as failure to recover consciousness following a course of ECT, as occurred in 2 patients in the present series.

The subacute onset of confusion accompanied by signs of focal brain disease is a common presentation of cerebral tumour and many patients with JCD are initially referred for neurosurgical opinion and investigation. Distinction may not be possible on clinical grounds before the appearance of more characteristic signs, in particular myoclonus. Conversely an intracranial neoplasm may closely imitate both the clinical and EEG findings of JCD. In my experience tumours in the region of the third ventricle or involving the corpus callosum have caused diagnostic difficulties, a further source of error being widespread dissemination of metastatic carcinoma.

At present of less practical importance but of great intrinsic interest is the distinction, where possible, from other 'degenerative' diseases. The clinical course of Alzheimer's disease is usually far more protracted, but in some patients the disease either progresses rapidly from the onset or appears to accelerate suddenly. In such patients myoclonus may be seen and the clinical differentiation from JCD becomes problematical. In one such patient I was able to study in detail each myoclonic jerk was accompanied by a spike discharge in the EEG, a finding not present in JCD. As Roos et al. (1973) point out, it is by no means certain that Alzheimer's disease and JCD are indeed entirely distinct, or that the former may not prove to be transmissible.

The clinical form of Parkinson's disease in which rigidity and dementia predominate also resembles the more chronic form of JCD and striatonigral degeneration is another source of difficulty. Progressive supranuclear palsy should be recognizable by the characteristic defects of ocular movements, but it is probable that the clinical manifestations of this disease have not yet been fully elucidated. There are undoubtedly other degenerative diseases, not yet classified as actual or potential clinicopathological entities, whose clinical features resemble those of JCD (Roos et al. 1973).

Motor neurone disease presents a particular problem. Anterior horn cell involvement and consequent severe muscle atrophy has long been recognized as a prominent feature in some patients with JCD. Dementia is occasionally seen in patients who both clinically and at autopsy are considered to have motor neurone disease. Claims that motor neurone disease is transmissible to primates have not been confirmed and there seems no doubt that the two diseases are distinct. From unavoidably limited experience I have tentatively concluded that a patient presenting with weakness and wasting who is mentally normal at the time will eventually be reported by the pathologist to have the changes of motor neurone disease even if dementia develops later. If dementia is obvious from an early stage of the disease (Allen et al. 1971), or is the presenting symptom, the pathology is likely to be that of JCD.

TREATMENT

From personal experince corticosteroids and corticotrophin have no effect on the course of JCD. Antiviral agents have been used without much rational basis. Amantadine has been reported as inducing partial remission (Braham 1971; Sanders & Dunn 1973) but no success was obtained in any patient in whom this agent was tried in the present series. Sanders and Dunn kindly allowed me to examine their Case 2 who may have recovered from the disease. When I saw her she was certainly normal but the original diagnosis must be considered uncertain. Idoxuridine has been tried without success (Goldhammer et al. 1972). It must be concluded that the concept of slow virus infection as a cause of JCD has not yet led to any therapeutic result.

ARE KURU AND JCD THE SAME DISEASE?

As kuru and JCD are the only two known human diseases considered to fulfil the criteria of slow virus infections it is natural to speculate on whether they might be the same disease modified by differing hosts. The possibility exists that one or more subjects with JCD or carrying the agent were eaten by their relatives in the highlands of New Guinea at some date between the probable introduction of cannibalism and the outbreak of the kuru epidemic. Alpers and Rail (1971) thought that two different agents were involved. The clinical details of human and experimental kuru differ in many respects from those of JCD. Kuru affected children of both sexes and adult women, but adult men were largely spared. This difference is almost certainly attributable, however, to differing exposure to cannibal feasts. Kuru appears to be far more stereotyped, an ataxic gait progressing to complete inability to walk, with tremor and pyramidal signs, and eventually dysarthria and dysphagia. It is not certain whether dementia is part of the clinical picture, whereas it is an invariable component of JCD. Myoclonus does not appear in either natural or experimental kuru although commonly present in both man and chimpanzee affected by JCD.

There have been several reports of a supposedly kuru-like disease in Europe and the USA. Seitelberger (1962) described a form of spinocerebellar degeneration accompanied by dementia occurring in middle age in several generations of a single family. The disease was progressive, leading to death in from 2 to 7 years. Pathological examination showed a systematized atrophy, mainly affecting the cerebellum and spinal cord, but with many senile plaques. Schaltenbrand et al. (1968) described the case of a boy who died at the age of 13 after an illness lasting $2\frac{1}{2}$ years and characterized by hyperkinesia, dystonia, ataxia and mental dulling. The autopsy showed slight spongy degeneration, neuronal loss maximal in the cerebellum and scanty PAS-positive plaques of the type seen in kuru. Horoupian et al. (1972) described a patient with clinical features typical of the subacute form of JCD, including myoclonus. The pathology was also that of JCD with the addition of numerous 'kuru plaques'. The specificity of these plaques has not been established and in the absence of any absolute diagnostic criteria the question of the possible identity of the two diseases cannot be satisfactorily answered.

THE EPIDEMIOLOGY OF JCD

The epidemiology of JCD must now be reconsidered with the aim of detecting any evidence of natural transmission. The disease is rare but has been reported from many European countries, from the USA, from Japan (Ishizaki et al. 1971) and from Israel, including immigrants from North Africa (Goldhammer et al. 1972). There are less reliable clinical reports from India (Omer 1964), Nigeria (Osuntokun 1971) and Chile (Rojas & Kase 1969).

Verified familial incidence is rare. In the Backer family (Jacob et al. 1950) members of 3 generations were clinically affected, with autopsy confirmation in 4 members in 2 generations. In the 'B' family (May et al. 1968) 3 generations also had the clinical features of the disease with autopsy confirmation in 3 members of the third generation. The 'R' family (Davison & Rabiner, 1940) are thought by most authorities to have had some different disease. Bonduelle et al. (1971) also described a family in which 3 generations appeared to be affected, with autopsy confirmation in 1 case, later confirmed as having the transmissible form of the disease. In these family studies, however, the emphasis is entirely on genetic factors, with no mention of matters of importance in a contagious disease, such as duration of contact of affected members.

There has been one confirmed example of conjugal JCD (Garzuly et al. 1971), both partners developing the disease simultaneously. Transmission from a common food source is by no means impossible. Brody (1973) conducted an epidemiological study on cases in the USA but found no convincing common factors. A remarkably high proportion of the patients had been in the habit of eating hogs' brains, but this was also a common practice among the controls. Transmission by direct contact must also be considered as in the laboratory both kuru and JCD can be transmitted by a vaccination scratch, admittedly using brain material.

My own study in England and Wales has not been completed and it is clear that full information will not be obtainable in many cases. There are inherent and perhaps insuperable difficulties in attempting to trace the source of infection in a disease which, if infectious at all, may have an incubation period of a decade or more. Information on possibly important matters, such as details of inoculations and illness in childhood, is often not available and the most that can be hoped for is that some factor or factors will be evident from the incomplete evidence obtained. As far as the information can be analysed it is clear that foreign travel has not been a factor, one woman indeed having lived all her life in the same house. Only one patient is known to have eaten brains; in the words of her mother, 'She was weaned on them'. No other dietary factor has seemed important. Two patients had had intracranial operations for trigeminal neuralgia, one 2 years before the onset of JCD and one at an interval not yet ascertained. In Nevin et al.'s (1960) series 2 of 8 patients had had cranial surgery. Serious head injury was not reported in any patient in the present series, although closed head injury has been reported as an antecedent factor (Behrman et al. 1962). No pattern of past illness could be detected. Only 1 patient is known to have had jaundice. In 2 patients diarrhoea and vomiting had immediately preceded or accompanied the onset of neurological symptoms. In 3 patients a near blood relative was said to have died of a similar disease but autopsy confirmation was not available.

Some contact with domestic pets, cats or dogs, was universal. The houses of 2 patients had been over-run with mice. One patient had close contact with a ferret and the husband of another patient had kept ferrets for many years up to 5 years before she developed the disease. A further patient had had some slight contact with ferrets as a child. In collaboration with Dr Malcolm Campbell and Dr Gajdusek it has been possible to initiate transmission experiments using the brain of the ferret that bit the first patient some 18 months before he developed symptoms of the disease. The ferret could possibly be a significant species in this context as the naturally occurring slow virus disease, mink encephalopathy, is transmissible to the ferret, but without producing fatal disease. The animal recovers but the agent is still present in the brain as it can be transmitted back to the mink

Transmissible and degenerative diseases

(Marsh et al. 1969). Needless to say, most patients have had no contact with ferrets or mink, alive or dead.

So far I have found evidence of one possible cluster of the disease in a small rural community. In 1964 a woman died of JCD, confirmed at autopsy. In 1967 a woman of 35, living 40 miles away, also died of the disease, subsequently shown to be the transmissible form. By chance I found that her sister, whom she visited frequently, lived one mile from the home of the first case. The sister's husband and the husband of the first woman to die were close friends. In 1971 a man living in the same group of small villages also died of the disease. He also knew the brother-in-law of the second case and worked for the same firm. I have not pursued this line of investigation further as there are obvious possibilities of causing fear and distress. The case material is being examined for other possible clusters but the difficulties of studying the epidemiology of this disease are illustrated by the fact that the relatives of the three patients described above were all quite ignorant of any possible contact.

I wish to acknowledge the help of the numerous physicians and pathologists who have allowed me to see their patients and records.

REFERENCES

Allen, I. V., Dermott, E., Connolly, J. H. & Hurwitz, L. J. (1971) A study of a patient with the amyotrophic form of Creutzfeldt–Jakob disease. *Brain*, 94, 715.

Alpers, M. & Rail, L. (1971) Kuru and Creutzfeldt–Jakob disease; clinical and aetiological aspects. *Proc. Aust. Ass. Neurol.*, 8, 7.

Behrman, S., Mandybur, T. & McMenemey, W. H. (1962) Un cas de maladie de Creuzfeld–Jacob (sic) à la suite d'un traumatisme cérébrale. *Rev. neurol.*, 107, 453.

Bonduelle, M., Escourolle, R., Bouyges, P., Lormeau, G., Ribadeau-Dumas, J.-L. & Merland, J.-J. (1971) Maladie de Creutzfeldt–Jakob familiale. Observation anatomo-clinique. *Rev. neurol.*, 125, 197.

Braham, J. (1971) Jakob–Creutzfeldt disease: treatment by amantadine. *Br. med. J.*, iv, 212.

Brody, J. A. (1973) Personal communication.

Brownell, B. & Oppenheimer, D. R. (1965) An ataxic form of subacute presenile polioencephalopathy (Creutzfeldt–Jakob disease). *J. Neurol. Neurosurg. Psychiat.*, 28, 350.

Clinical aspects of slow virus infections

Creutzfeldt, H. G. (1920) Über eine eingenartige herdförmige Erkrankung des Zentralnervensystems. *Z. ges. Neurol. Psychiat.*, **57**, 1.

Davison, C. & Rabiner, A. M. (1940) Spastic pseudosclerosis. *Archs Neurol. Psychiat., Chicago*, **19**, 573.

Von Economo, C. & Schilder, P. (1920) Über einer Pseudosclerose nahestehende Erkrankung im Präsenium. *Z. ges. Neurol. Psychiat.*, **55**, 1.

Gajdusek, D. C. & Gibbs, C. J. (1972) Transmission of kuru from man to rhesus monkey (*Macaca mulatta*) 8½ years after inoculation. *Nature, Lond.*, **240**, 351.

Gajdusek, D. C., Gibbs, C. J. & Alpers, M. (1966) Experimental transmission of a kuru-like syndrome to chimpanzees. *Nature, Lond.*, **209**, 794.

Garzuly, F., Jellinger, K. & Pilz, P. (1971) Subakute spongiöse Encephalopathie (Jakob–Creutzfeldt Syndrom). Klinisch-morphologische Analyse von 9 Fällen. *Arch. Psychiat. NervKrankh.*, **214**, 207.

Gibbs, C. J. & Gajdusek, D. C. (1972) Transmission of scrapie to the cynomolgus monkey (*Macaca fascicularis*). *Nature, Lond.*, **236**, 73.

Gibbs, C. J., Gajdusek, D. C., Asher, P. M., Alpers, M. P., Beck, E., Daniel, P. M. & Matthews, W. B. (1968) Creutzfeldt–Jakob disease (spongiform encephalopathy): transmission to the chimpanzee. *Science, N.Y.*, **161**, 388.

Goldhammer, Y., Bubis, J. J., Sarovapinhas, I. & Braham, J. (1972) Subacute spongiform encephalopathy and its relation to Jakob–Creutzfeldt disease: report on 6 cases. *J. Neurol. Neurosurg. Psychiat.*, **35**, 1.

Heidenhain, A. (1929) Klinische und anatomische Untersuchungen über eine eigenartige organische Erkrankung des Zentralnervensystems im Praesenium. *Z. ges. Neurol. Psychiat.*, **118**, 49.

Horoupian, D. S., Powers, J. M. & Schaumberg, H. H. (1972) Kuru-like neuropathological changes in a North American. *Archs Neurol., Chicago*, **27**, 555.

Ishizaki, T., Fukase, K. & Kashimura, H. (1971) An intermediate case between Creutzfeldt–Jakob disease and subacute spongiform encephalopathy. Report of an autopsy case. *Clin. Neurol.*, **11**, 601.

Jacob, H., Pyrkosch, W. & Strube, H. (1950) Die erbliche Form der Creutzfeldt–Jakobschen Krankheit. *Arch. Psychiat. NervKrankh.*, **184**, 653.

Jakob, A. (1921a) Über eigenartige Erkankungen des Zentranervensystems mit bemerkswertem anatomischem Befunde (spastische Pseudosklerose-Encephalomyelopathie mit disseminierten Degenerationsherden). *Z. ges. Neurol. Psychiat.*, **64**, 147.

Jakob, A. (1921b) Über eine der multiplen Sklerose klinisch nahestehende Erkrankung des Zentralnervensystems (spastische Pseudoskerlose) mit bemerkswertem anatomischem Befunde. *Med. Klin.*, **17**, 372.

Jones, D. P. & Nevin, S. (1954) Rapidly progressive cerebral degeneration (subacute vascular encephalopathy) with mental disorder, focal disturbances and myoclonic epilepsy. *J. Neurol. Neurosurg. Psychiat.*, **17**, 148.

Kirschbaum, W. R. (1968) *Jakob–Creutzfeldt Disease*. New York: Elsevier.

Marsh, R. F., Burger, D., Eckroade, R., Zu Rhein, G. M. & Hanson, R. P. (1969) A preliminary report on the experimental host range of the transmissible mink encephalopathy agent. *J. infect. Dis.*, **120**, 713.

May, W. W., Itabashi, H. H. & Dejong, R. N. (1968) Creutzfeldt–Jakob disease. II. Clinical pathologic and genetic study of a family. *Archs Neurol., Chicago*, **19**, 137.

Nevin, S., Barnard, R. O. & McMenemey, W. H. (1967) Different types of Creutzfeldt–Jakob disease. *Acta neuropath.*, Suppl. III, 7.

Nevin, S., McMenemey, W. H., Behrman, S. & Jones, D. P. (1960) Subacute spongiform encephalopathy. A subacute form of encephalopathy attributable to vascular dysfunction (spongiform cerebral atrophy). *Brain*, **83**, 519.

Omer, S. (1964) Jakob–Creutzfeldt syndrome. *J. Indian med. Ass.*, **43**, 398.

Osuntokun, B. O. (1971) The pattern of neurological illness in tropical Africa. Experience at Ibadan, Nigeria. *J. neurol. Sci.*, **12**, 417.

Rojas, G. & Kase, J. C. (1969) Sindrome de Haidenhain. Presentación de un cas. *Neurocirugía, Santiago*, **27**, 110.

Roos, R., Gajdusek, D. C. & Gibbs, C. J. (1973) The clinical characteristics of transmissible Creutzfeldt–Jakob disease. *Brain*, **96**, 1.

Van Rossum, A. (1968) Spastic pseudosclerosis (Creutzfeldt–Jakob disease). In *Handbook of Clinical Neurology*, ed. Vinken, P. J. & Bruyn, G. W. vol. 6, pp. 726–60. Amsterdam: North Holland.

Sanders, W. L. & Dunn, T. L. (1973) Creutzfeldt–Jakob disease treated with amantidine (*sic*). *J. Neurol. Neurosurg. Psychiat.*, **36**, 581.

Schaltenbrand, G., Trosdorf, E., Orthner, H. & Henn, R. (1968) Kuruähnliche sklerosende Panencephalomyelitis in Europa. *Dt. Z. NervHeilk.*, **193**, 158.

Seitelberger, F. (1962) Eigenartige familiär-hereditäre Krankheit des Zentralnervensystems in einer niederösterreichischen Sippe. *Wien. klin. Wschr.*, **74**, 687.

10

Pathology of Transmissible and Degenerative Diseases of the Nervous System

D. R. OPPENHEIMER

The chapters in this section are concerned with four diseases, two of which—scrapie in sheep and encephalopathy in mink—are not known to affect human beings. The other two—kuru and the condition which some call subacute spongiform encephalopathy and others Jakob–Creutzfeldt disease—are not known to occur in other animals except as a result of inoculation. The common features of these four are:

1. They are all progressive, and generally fatal, diseases running a subacute course and affecting mainly or exclusively the grey matter of the central nervous system.

2. The histopathology of the brain in these four diseases is similar in its main features, and resembles that of the diseases which are commonly called 'degenerative' rather than that of the proved virus infections of the brain.

3. The injection into some species of animal of an extract of brain or other visceral tissues from an affected individual gives rise, after a long interval, to a progressive disease which resembles the 'natural' disease both in clinical and in histological details.

4. The 'agents' or substances responsible for the animal transmissions have up to now defied efforts at chemical, electron-

microscopical or immunological characterization.

The large amount of research on these conditions during the last 15 years has given rise to a volcanic eruption of publications, including a number of symposia and review articles (Gajdusek et al. 1965; Field 1969; Whitty et al. 1969; Thormar 1971; Dick 1972; Lampert et al. 1972).

The obvious questions waiting for an answer are: first, what sort of things these transmissible agents may be, and how they do their deadly work; second, what part, if any, the agents play in the causation of the naturally occurring diseases; third, what is the nature of the so-called degenerative diseases of the central nervous system; and fourth, whether a transmissible agent is involved in the pathology of other degenerative conditions. A further major problem is that of genetic transmission in the experimentally transmissible diseases. In the case of scrapie, there is impressive statistical evidence (Parry 1962) of transmission by a single autosomal recessive gene. Whether the natural disease is ever acquired by infection in the field is still a matter of dispute (Dickinson et al. 1965; Brotherston et al. 1968; Parry 1969). Kuru was originally thought (Bennett et al. 1959) to be genetically determined, but the evidence was inconclusive because the facts about parenthood in the Fore tribe were hard to collect. Later, it seemed probable that ritual cannibalism was the main factor in the spread of the disease (Glasse 1967), but a genetic factor has not been excluded (Gajdusek & Alpers 1972). In spongiform encephalopathy, which is usually a sporadic disease, a few families are described in which the disease appears to be transmitted as an autosomal dominant (Davison & Rabiner 1940; Friede & DeJong 1964; Kirschbaum 1968; May et al. 1968). Now that transmission to primates from two familial cases has been achieved (Roos et al. 1973) it is no longer reasonable to regard genetic transmission and infection as mutually exclusive mechanisms in the pathology of these diseases. Parry (1962) clearly stated the problem in relation to scrapie, and offered a theoretical model; but up to the present there is no generally accepted theory of how a disease may be at the same time genetically determined and experimentally transmissible.

The answers to these questions will not be provided by conventional histopathology, but it is worth recalling that it was the observation of histological similarities between scrapie and kuru (Hadlow 1959) that led to the discovery of transmissible degenerative diseases in man. Similarities and differences between histological appearances are no more than suggestive clues to similarities and differences between basic pathological processes, but they may serve as a check on light-hearted speculation. For example, the histological differences between a degenerative and a demyelinating disease are so great that it is well-nigh impossible to suppose that they have a common pathological basis. In what follows, the histological features of a number of 'degenerative' conditions will be summarized, and compared with those of scrapie, kuru and Jakob's encephalopathy, both natural and experimental. Mink encephalopathy will not be discussed. From published accounts (Burger & Hartsough 1965; Hartsough & Burger 1965; Barlow 1972) it seems to resemble scrapie very closely, both clinically and histologically, except that there is no conclusive evidence of either vertical or horizontal transmission of the 'natural' disease. Both these conditions are discussed elsewhere in this book.

The degenerative diseases are those in which, for reasons of which we are ignorant, nerve cells and their processes shrivel, die and disappear in a more or less symmetrical and systemic manner. However they are caused, they seem to be totally distinct from, for instance, the demyelinating diseases, in which the obvious damage is to myelin sheaths rather than to nerve cells or their processes: from vascular or biochemical disorders, in which cells suffer from metabolic deprivation: from the lipidoses and leucodystrophies, in which abnormal substances pile up in brain tissue, apparently as a result of enzyme deficiencies: and from acute or subacute inflammatory processes, due either to the presence in the brain and cord of an identifiable pathogenic organism, or to an abnormal immunological response. Difficulties may, however, arise in the histological distinction between a 'degenerative' condition and some effects of exogenous poisoning (in particular poisoning by heavy metals), of endogenous poisoning in some liver diseases, or of malignant disease (for instance, carcinomatous degeneration of the cerebellar cortex).

The common feature of the degenerative diseases is a 'spontaneous', i.e. unexplained, loss of nerve cells in particular sites. Table 13 shows the sites at which cell loss is observed in a few of the commoner types of degenerative disease. The general rule is that in any one disease a few, or many, sites are at risk, but in an individual case only a selection of these may be affected. In motor neurone disease there is progressive loss of motor cells at all levels of the brainstem and spinal cord, but sparing the oculomotor nuclei. In most cases this is accompanied by a 'dying-back' of the pyramidal tracts; that is, the loss of pyramidal fibres is always more severe at lower than at higher levels (Brownell et al. 1970). This 'dying-back' phenomenon is seen in the pyramidal and other fibre tracts in a number of degenerative diseases, including some cases of Jakob's encephalopathy. Paralysis agitans affects primarily the pigmented cells of the brain stem, and in some cases the autonomic efferent cells of the brain stem and cord (Bannister & Oppenheimer 1972). In the kind of multiple system atrophy, either sporadic or familial, which includes olivopontocerebellar and striatonigral degeneration, a large number of cell groups are at risk, and individual cases show degeneration in various selections of these (Bannister & Oppenheimer 1972). In Friedreich's ataxia many cell groups are affected, including sensory ganglion cells (Hughes et al. 1968). The list of structures at risk in classical Friedreich's ataxia shows little overlap with the list in multiple system atrophy; there are, however, very numerous recorded cases, both sporadic and familial, of unclassifiable degenerations of the cerebellar and other systems, which overlap with both multiple system atrophy and Friedreich's ataxia. The most notable instance is a family studied by Schut and Haymaker (1951) in which a single dominant gene appears to have been responsible for an astonishing variety of clinical syndromes and anatomical lesions. In Huntington's disease the striatum (caudate nucleus and putamen) is affected, and to a lesser degree the cerebral cortex. In kuru and Jakob's encephalopathy multiple sites are again at risk (Fowler & Robertson 1959; Klatzo et al.

TABLE 13

SITES OF NEURONAL LOSS IN VARIOUS DEGENERATIVE CONDITIONS

Site	Motor neurone disease	Paralysis agitans	Multiple system atrophy	Friedreich's ataxia	Huntington's disease	Kuru	Jakob's encephalopathy
Cortex	(+)	-	(+)	-	+	+	+ +
Striatum	-	(+)	+	-	+ +	+	+
Pallidum	-	-	(+)	(+)	+ +	-	(+)
Thalamus	-	-	(+)	-	-	+	+
Hypothalamus	-	+	-	-	-	+	+
Pigmented nuclei	-	+ +	+	-	-	+	-
Pontine nuclei	-	-	+	-	-	+	-
Inferior olives	-	-	+	-	-	+	-
Dorsal vagal nuclei	-	(+)	+	-	-	-	-
Purkinje cells	-	-	(+)	-	-	+	(+)
Granule cells	-	-	-	-	-	+	+
Dentate nuclei	-	-	-	+ +	-	(+)	(+)
Motor cells	+ +	-	(+)	(+)	-	?	+
Intermediolateral	-	(+)	-	-	-	?	-
Sensory ganglia	-	-	-	+ +	-	-	-
Optic nerves	-	-	-	+	-	+	-
Pyramidal tracts	+	-	+	+ +	-	+	+
Spinocerebellar tracts	(+)	-	(+)	+ +	-	+	-

+ + Always or nearly always affected
+ Commonly affected
(+) Occasionally affected
- Seldom if ever affected

1969; Kirschbaum 1968; Beck et al. 1969) in particular the cerebral cortex, striatum, thalamus and cerebellar cortex. There is considerable overlap between the two; the emphasis in kuru tends to be on the cerebellum and in Jakob's disease on the cerebrum, but there is a group of cases of Jakob's disease in which cerebellar cortical lesions predominate (Brownell & Oppenheimer 1965).

Special histological features, other than neuronal loss and resultant gliosis, are associated with various degenerative diseases. For instance, there are the Lewy inclusion bodies, which are seen mainly in the pigmented cells in cases of paralysis agitans. They are not associated with any other disease, though they are occasionally present as incidental findings in the brains of elderly subjects. In Alzheimer's disease, in addition to cell loss in the cerebral cortex there are characteristic changes (neurofibrillary tangles and granulovacuolar degeneration) in cortical cells, and argyrophilic/congophilic 'plaques' in the cortex. In kuru also, and occasionally in natural scrapie, there are characteristic plaques (Plate VII/1) of amyloid material, seen most frequently in the cerebellar cortex. In spongiform encephalopathy, there are areas of status spongiosus in the cerebral cortex (Plate VII/2); and in scrapie, there are conspicuous vacuoles in the cytoplasm of some types of nerve cell, especially in the brainstem (Plate VII/3). Similar vacuoles are present in human kuru, but are not seen in the experimental disease (Beck et al. 1969). Status spongiosus is found in both human and experimental kuru, and in experimental scrapie, but not in natural scrapie (Beck et al. 1969). Finally there have been four reports (Chou & Martin 1971; Horoupian et al. 1972; Krücke et al. 1973; Adams et al. 1974) of the finding of so-called kuru plaques in sporadic cases from North America and Britain, diagnosed clinically as cases of Jakob's encephalopathy (Plate VIII/1). These overlaps are summarized in Table 14.

It is clear that these 6 conditions—scrapie, kuru and spongiform encephalopathy, and their experimental counterparts—have a great deal in common, histologically as well as in other respects. There is also some blurring of outlines between this group of diseases and other degenerative conditions. One may, for instance,

TABLE 14

SPECIAL FEATURES OF SCRAPIE, KURU AND
JAKOB'S ENCEPHALOPATHY

Disease	*Status spongiosus*	*Vacuoles in nerve cells*	*PAS-positive plaques*
Scrapie			
Natural	−	+ +	+
Experimental (mice)	+	+	+
Kuru			
Natural	+	+	+
Experimental	+ +	−	−
Jakob's encephalopathy			
Natural	+	(+)	(+)
Experimental	+	+	−

+ + Always or nearly always occur
  + commonly occur
(+) Occasionally occur
  − Seldom if ever occur

find status spongiosus indistinguishable from that seen in Jakob's encephalopathy, in an otherwise typical case of Alzheimer's disease, or in a case of motor neurone disease without dementia (Plate VIII/1, 2). Conversely, the spinal cords of some cases of Jakob's encephalopathy show the characteristic changes of motor neurone disease, and nothing else.

Turning to the astrocytic hyperplasia which has attracted so much attention in this group of diseases, it is a general principle that any sort of damage to central nervous tissues, short of complete stoppage of the blood supply, is followed by hypertrophy and proliferation of astrocytes. This reaction is seen in plaques of demyelination, or surrounding areas of trauma, infarction or haemorrhage, in cerebral oedema, in 'toxic' encephalopathies, and of course in areas of neuronal degeneration. Wherever nerve cells die, astrocytic gliosis ensues. In the degenerative diseases, it is usually taken for granted that the observed gliosis is simply the result of nerve cell loss or damage, and does not imply a primary derangement of astrocytic functions. In Jakob's encephalopathy, on the other hand, it has frequently been observed that the degree of astrocytic hyperplasia in a particular site appears to be out of all proportion to the loss of nerve cells, and has even been present throughout the grey matter of the brain and spinal cord, whereas loss of nerve cells is restricted to a few sites. It has long been suspected that the disease is a primary affliction of the glia. This view has not been disproved, but it is worth remembering, firstly, that neuronal loss may be very difficult to assess, apart from 'easy' situations such as the hippocampus or the cerebellar cortex; and secondly, that astrocytes react in their usual manner not only where neuronal bodies are lost, but also when the terminal fibres in a particular area have degenerated—for instance, degeneration in the posterior columns of the spinal cord gives rise to an intense gliosis, without cell loss, in the gracile and cuneate nuclei. The reaction of astrocytes to degeneration of axon terminals in a similar situation has been demonstrated experimentally by Illis (1973). The same principle has been invoked (Brownell et al. 1970) to explain the finding, in many cases of motor neurone disease, of an intense astrocytic hyperplasia in the thalamus and striatum, without detectable loss of nerve cells. Thus if one sees an abnormal proliferation of astrocytes in an otherwise normal-looking hippocampus in a case of Jakob's disease (Plate VIII/3) one cannot infer that the astrocytes are behaving abnormally without first ascertaining whether there is a normal number of terminal axons entering the hippocampus; and this would be a difficult task. In other words, great caution is needed in the interpretation of an apparently primary hyperplasia or hypertrophy of astrocytes.

This is not to deny the possibility that malfunction or neuroglia may be the primary event in some of the neuronal degenerations. Many functions have been ascribed to astrocytes. Of these, two seem to be well established. The first is that of laying down glial fibres in damaged areas. Astrocytes undoubtedly do this, though the biological usefulness of the procedure is not very obvious. The second function is the nutrition of nerve cells. The evidence for this is largely morphological, and based on the fact that neurones have no direct contact with capillaries, whereas astrocytes have close contacts with both neurones and capillaries. As far

PLATE VII

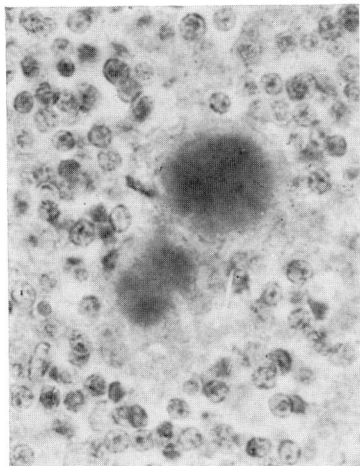

Fig. 1. 'Kuru plaques': two plaques from the cerebellar cortex of a kuru patient. There is a central core of PAS-positive material, surrounded by a fibrillar corona. The surrounding nuclei are of cerebellar granule cells.

Periodic acid Schiff. × 70

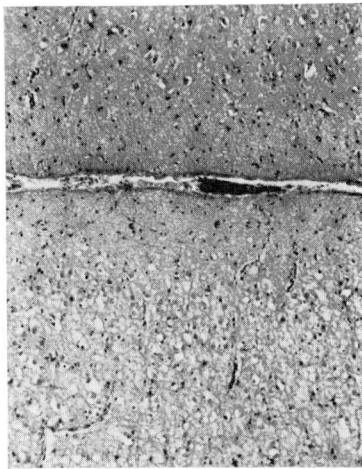

Fig. 2. Status spongiosus in Jakob's encephalopathy. The cortex in the lower part of the picture is severely affected; that on the other side of the sulcus shows merely artefactual spaces due to the embedding process.

Phosphotungstic acid haematoxylin. × 56

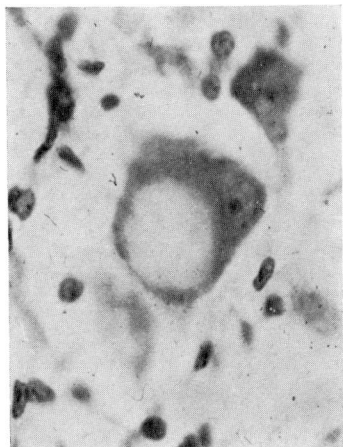

Fig. 3. A vacuolated nerve cell in natural scrapie.

Nissl. × 900

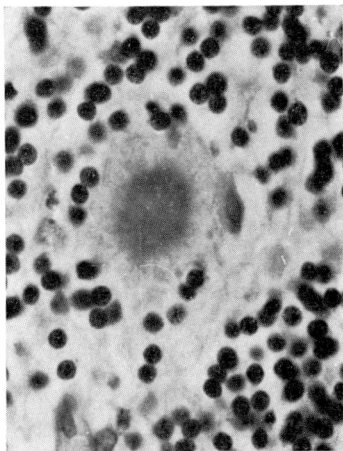

Fig. 4. A 'kuru plaque' from the cerebellar cortex of a patient suffering from Jakob's encephalopathy.

Periodic acid Schiff. × 630

PLATE VIII

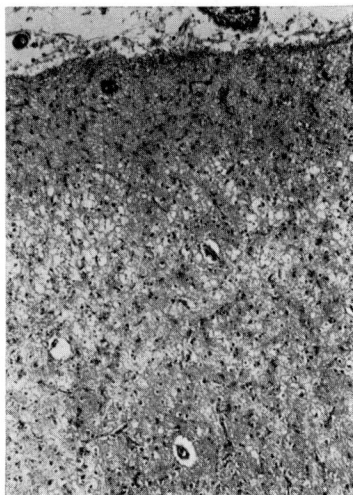

Fig. 1. Status spongiosus in a patient suffering from Alzheimer's disease. Argyrophilic plaques and neurofibrillary tangles were present in the same area.

Phosphotungstic acid haematoxylin. × 56

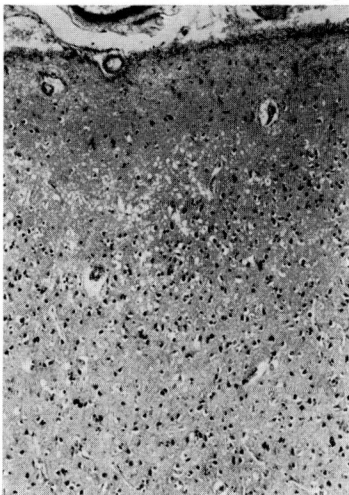

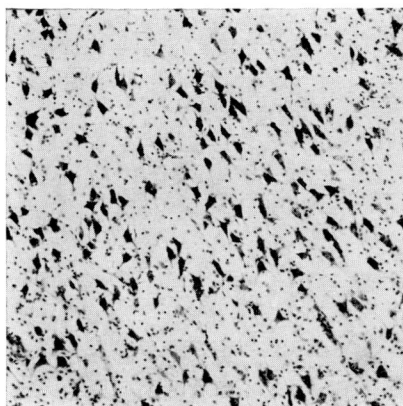

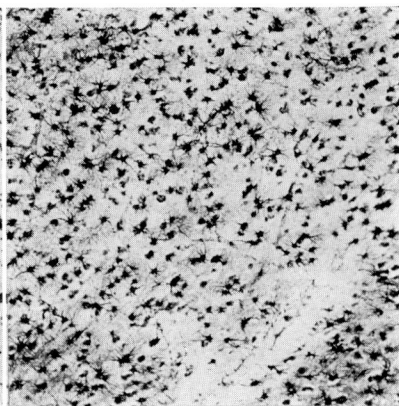

Fig. 2. Status spongiosus in a patient suffering from motor neurone disease.

Phosphotungstic acid haematoxylin. × 56

Fig. 3. The end-folium of the hippocampus in a patient suffering from Jakob's encephalopathy. (*a*) A normal population of nerve cells. (*b*) Intense astrocytic proliferation.

(*a*) *Nissl.* × 660
(*b*) *Cajal's gold impregnation.* × 660

as is known, individual astrocytes in grey matter perform both functions: and it is a plausible theory (Field 1969) that an astrocyte which has been stimulated to divide, swell and lay down glial fibres may tend to neglect its duties as a wet-nurse. Whether astrocytes in white matter have the same metabolic obligations towards axis cylinders, or whether the axons are entirely fed by their parent cell bodies, is not known. In either case, astrocytic inadequacy might be the immediate cause of the 'dying-back' phenomenon, and eventually of neuronal loss. Unfortunately, there is at present no sure way of distinguishing between a primary disorder of neurones and a secondary deficiency due to glial inadequacy. Histochemical study of biopsies from cases of Jakob's encephalopathy (Friede & DeJong 1964) have shown a lack of oxidative enzymes in nerve cells, but not in astrocytes. Electron microscopy studies of biopsies from areas of status spongiosus (Gonatas et al. 1965; Bignami & Forno 1970) have shown abnormal vacuoles in the processes of both neurones and astrocytes, but these findings do not settle the question.

However attractive the idea of glial inadequacy may be in the context of degenerative diseases, there is very little to be said in its favour when applied to other conditions, such as trauma and infarction, in which astrocytic activity is observed. In multiple sclerosis, for instance, the earliest changes are seen in myelin sheaths: these are followed by microglial proliferation and often by lymphocytic cuffing of small veins. Astrocytic hypertrophy is seen at a later stage, is restricted to the vicinity of the lesion, and is reasonably regarded as purely reactive. There is no reason, here, to suspect that the astrocytes are neglecting their metabolic functions; a multiple sclerosis lesion in grey matter may be swarming with astrocytes, but the nerve cell bodies in the plaque appear to be in perfect health.

A word is needed about the nomenclature of the condition commonly referred to as Jakob–Creutzfeldt disease (see Kirschbaum (1968) for references). Jakob in 1921 and 1923 described the clinical and pathological features of 5 cases of subacute progressive multifocal degeneration of cerebral and spinal grey matter. The patients were aged between 34 and 52 years, and the disease lasted between 6 and 15 months. Jakob considered that the case, described by Creutzfeldt in 1920, of a girl dying at the age of 23 after an episodic illness lasting 18 months, was of a similar type. Creutzfeldt himself disagreed with this, and it is doubtful whether any modern neurologist (or neuropathologist) would make the diagnosis of Jakob's encephalopathy if he were presented with Creutzfeldt's case. It would not be unfair to Creutzfeldt's shade if his name were omitted in this context. The question then arises whether or not the condition described by Jakob is a single disease, and if so whether it is the same as the one described by Nevin (1970) and Nevin et al. (1960) under the name of subacute spongiform encephalopathy. Professor Matthews in an earlier chapter refers to his inability to distinguish between the two from their clinical features and it is difficult to apply the principles by which Nevin distinguishes the histopathology of spongiform encephalopathy from that of Jakob's disease. The differences that may be seen between one case and another appear to be either differences in local intensity of the disease, or such as are readily explicable in terms of the time course of the degenerative process.

A convincing method of differentiating between the two conditions, if in fact they are different, would be the demonstration that one of them is transmissible, the other not. According to a recent report from the Bethesda workers (Roos et al. 1973) all patients from whom successful animal inoculations have been made fall into the spongiform encephalopathy group; results are still awaited from two cases of (by Nevin's criteria) Jakob's disease. An addendum to the same paper, however, refers to a successful transmission from an Oxford case, in which, in addition to the cerebral changes, there were well-marked changes typical of motor neurone disease in the spinal cord, and which at the time was regarded as satisfying Nevin's criteria for a diagnosis of Jakob's disease. The question whether Jakob's disease (as opposed to spongiform encephalopathy) is a single entity, or merely part of a broad continuum of system degenerations, which includes motor neurone disease, Huntington's disease and olivopontocerebellar atrophy, as Nevin suggests, is one which cannot be settled at present. Kirschbaum (1968), who does not accept Nevin's view that spongiform encephalopathy is a distinct entity, appears to be confused on the subject. Much of what he writes seems to be based on the idea that Jakob–Creutzfeldt disease is an entity, with variable clinical and pathological features, but towards the end of his book he states that the syndrome merely represents a particular kind of tissue response to a wide variety of causative agents. This view is justified if one accepts all the 150 cases listed by Kirschbaum as examples of the same syndrome; but it is likely that a number of these, including Creutzfeldt's case, would be thrown out of the discussion by Professor Matthews and by most neuropathologists. These questions remain unsettled. Meanwhile, it is suggested that spongiform encephalopathy should be classified together with the syndrome described by Jakob under the single heading of *Jakob's encephalopathy*.

About four years ago Daniel (1971), speaking on this subject, pleaded eloquently for an open-minded approach to the problem of how a slowly-developing, non-inflammatory degenerative disease of the nervous system could at the same time be genetically determined (as in the case of scrapie) and be experimentally transmissible by a replicating agent. Since that time the most significant development has been the animal transmission of the disease from two familial cases of Jakob's encephalopathy (Roos et al. 1973). It is, of course, conceivable that infection within a family group might give a false impression of a genetic disease with dominant inheritance; but this theory has not been seriously maintained in the case of the famous Backer family, with its six or more cases of Jakob's encephalopathy in three generations (Kirschbaum 1968).

There has been one report (Jellinger et al. 1972) indicating that Jakob's encephalopathy may be acquired by natural infection. The report concerned a married couple, in both of whom the disease was demonstrated histologically. More recently, there has been a report (Duffy et al. 1974) suggesting artificial transmission in man. Here, the disease developed 18 months after receiving a corneal graft taken from a patient dying of Jakob's encephalopathy. Again, the diagnosis was confirmed histologically in both donor and recipient. In view of the rarity of the disease, it is very unlikely that these are examples of pure coincidence.

In the past, it has often been assumed that where a transmissible agent has been demonstrated, the natural disease is necessarily caused by infection. This assumption has led many workers on scrapie to ignore the evidence for genetic transmission of the natural disease. I should like to express vigorous agreement with Professor Daniel, not only in supporting his plea for open-mindedness, but also in deprecating the use of the term 'slow virus infection' and the tendency to force other diseases of un-known aetiology, with a manifestly different pathology from that of scrapie, kuru and Jakob's encephalopathy, into the same category.

REFERENCES

Adams, H., Beck, E. & Shenkin, A. M. (1974) Creutzfeldt–Jakob disease: further similarities with Kuru. *J. Neurol. Neurosurg. Psychiat.*, **37**, 195.

Bannister, R. & Oppenheimer, D. R. (1972) Degenerative diseases of the nervous system associated with autonomic failure. *Brain*, **95**, 457.

Barlow, R. M. (1972) Transmissible mink encephalopathy: pathogenesis and nature of the aetiological agent. *J. clin. Path.*, **25**, suppl. 6, 102.

Beck, E., Daniel, P. M., Gajdusek, D. C. & Gibbs, C. J. (1969) Similarities and differences in the pattern of the pathological changes in scrapie, kuru, experimental kuru and subacute presenile polioencephalopathy. In *Virus Diseases and the Nervous System*, ed. Whitty, C. W. M., Hughes, J. T. & MacCallum, F. O., pp. 107–20. Oxford: Blackwell Scientific.

Bennett, J. H., Rhodes, F. A. & Robson, H. N. (1959) A possible genetic basis for kuru. *Am. J. hum. Genet.*, **11**, 169.

Bignami, A. & Forno, L. S. (1970) Status spongiosus in Jakob–Creutz-feldt disease. *Brain*, **93**, 89.

Brotherston, J. G., Renwick, C. C., Stamp, J. T. & Zlotnik, I. (1968) Spread of scrapie by contact to goats and sheep. *J. comp. Path.*, **78**, 9.

Brownell, B. & Oppenheimer, D. R. (1965) An ataxic form of subacute presenile polioencephalopathy. *J. Neurol. Neurosurg. Psychiat.*, **28**, 350.

Brownell, B., Oppenheimer, D. R. & Hughes, J. T. (1970) The central nervous system in motor neurone disease. *J. Neurol. Neurosurg. Psychiat.*, **33**, 338.

Burger, D. & Hartsough, G. R. (1965) Encephalopathy of mink: II. Experimental and natural transmission. *J. infect. Dis.*, **115**, 393.
Chou, S. M. & Martin, J. D. (1971) Kuru-plaques in a case of Creutz-feldt–Jakob disease. *Acta neuropath.*, **17**, 150.
Daniel, P. M. (1971) Transmissible degenerative diseases of the nervous system. *Proc. R. Soc. Med.*, **64**, 787.
Davison, C. & Rabiner, A. M. (1940) Spastic pseudosclerosis. *Archs Neurol. Psychiat.*, *Chicago*, **44**, 578.
Dick, G. (1972) Host-virus reactions with special reference to persistent agents. *J. clin. Path.*, **25**, Suppl. 6.
Dickinson, A. G., Young, G. B., Stamp, J. T. & Renwick, C. C. (1965) An analysis of natural scrapie in Suffolk sheep. *Heredity*, **20**, 485.
Duffy, P., Wolf, J., Collins, G., DeVoe, A. G., Streeten, B. & Cowen, D. (1974) Possible person-to-person transmission of Creutzfeldt–Jakob disease (letter). *New Engl. J. Med.*, **290**, 692.
Field, E. J. (1969) Slow virus infections of the nervous system. *Int. Rev. exp. Path.*, **8**, 129.
Fowler, M. & Robertson, E. G. (1959) Observations on Kuru. III. Pathological features in five cases. *Aust. Ann. Med.*, **8**, 16.
Friede, R. L. & DeJong, R. N. (1964) Neuronal enzymatic failure in Creutzfeldt–Jakob disease (a familial study). *Archs Neurol.*, *Chicago*, **10**, 181.
Gajdusek, D. C. & Alpers, M. (1972) Genetic studies in relation to Kuru. *Am. J. hum. Genet.*, **24**, Suppl. S1.
Gajdusek, D. C., Gibbs, C. J. & Alpers, M. (1965) *Slow, Latent and Temperate Virus infections.* NINDB Monograph No. 2. U.S. Department of Health, Education and Welfare.
Glasse, R. M. (1967) Cannibalism in the kuru region of New Guinea. *Trans. N.Y. Acad. Sci.*, **29**, 748.
Gonatas, N. K., Terry, R. D. & Weiss, M. (1965) Electronmicroscopic study in two cases of Jakob–Creutzfeldt disease. *J. Neuropath. exp. Neurol.*, **24**, 575.
Hadlow, W. J. (1959) Scrapie and kuru. *Lancet*, **ii**, 289.
Hartsough, G. R. & Burger, D. (1965) Encephalopathy of mink: I. Epizootiologic and clinical observations. *J. infect. Dis.*, **115**, 387.
Horoupian, D. S., Powers, J. M. & Schaumburg, H. H. (1972) Kuru-like neuropathological changes in a North American. *Archs Neurol.*, *Chicago*, **27**, 555.
Hughes, J. T., Brownell, B. & Hewer, R. L. (1968) The peripheral sensory pathway in Friedreich's ataxia. *Brain*, **91**, 803.
Illis, L. S. (1973) Experimental model of regeneration in the central nervous system: II. The reaction of glia in the synaptic zone. *Brain*, **96**, 61.
Jellinger, K., Seitelberger, F., Heiss, W. D. & Holczabek, W. (1972) Konjugale Form der subakuten spongiösen Enzephalopathie. *Wien. klin. Wschr.*, **84**, 245.
Kirschbaum, W. R. (1968) *Jakob-Creutzfeldt Disease.* Amsterdam: Elsevier.

Klatzo, I., Gajdusek, D. C. & Zigas, V. (1959) Pathology of kuru. *Lab. Invest.*, **8,** 799.

Krücke, W., Beck, E. & Vitzthum, H. (1973) Creutzfeldt–Jakob disease: some unusual morphological features reminiscent of Kuru. *Z. Neurol.*, **206,** 1.

Lampert, P. W., Gajdusek, D. C. & Gibbs, C. J. (1972) Subacute spongiform virus encephalopathies. *Am. J. Path.*, **68,** 626.

May, W. W., Itabashi, H. H. & DeJong, R. N. (1968) Creutzfeldt–Jakob disease: clinical, pathologic and genetic study of a family. *Archs Neurol., Chicago*, **19,** 137.

Nevin, S. (1967) On some aspects of cerebral degeneration in later life. *Proc. R. Soc. Med.*, **60,** 517.

Nevin, S., McMenemey, W. H., Behrman, S. & Jones, D. P. (1960) Subacute spongiform encephalopathy. *Brain*, **83,** 519.

Parry, H. B. (1962) Scrapie: a transmissible and hereditary disease of sheep. *Heredity*, **17,** 75.

Parry, H. B. (1969) Scrapie—natural and experimental. In *Virus Diseases and the Nervous System*, ed. Whitty, C. W. M., Hughes, J. T. & MacCallum, F. O., pp. 99–105. Oxford: Blackwell Scientific.

Roos, R., Gajdusek, D. C. & Gibbs, C. J. (1973) The clinical characteristics of transmissible Creutzfeldt–Jakob disease. *Brain*, **96,** 1.

Schut, J. W. & Haymaker, W. (1951) Hereditary ataxia: a pathological study of five cases of common ancestry. *J. Neuropath. clin. Neurol.*, **1,** 183.

Thormar, H. (1971) Slow infections of the central nervous system. *Z. Neurol.*, **199,** 1–23, 151.

Whitty, C. W. M., Hughes, J. T. & MacCallum, F. O. (1969) *Virus Diseases and the Nervous System*. Oxford: Blackwell Scientific.

11

*Transmission Experiments and Degenerative
Conditions of the Central Nervous System*

E. J. FIELD

The modern study of slow infection of the central nervous system
derives from 3 seminal lectures delivered in the University of
London in 1954 by the late Dr Bjørn Sigurdsson, then director of
the Keldur Institute, Reykjavik. In these Sigurdsson (1954)
described certain naturally occurring diseases of sheep in Iceland
which had seemingly followed the importation of 20 Karakul
sheep from Halle in Germany in 1933. One disease he described
was maedi (which in Icelandic means dyspnoea or breathlessness)
—a slowly evolving pneumonitis in which the lungs develop a
rubbery consistency. It is now known to be due to an organism
very similar to, if indeed not identical with, that producing a
slowly progressive disease of the brain in sheep known as visna.
This latter, at first thought to be a 'demyelinating' disease, is now
recognized as a periventicular granulomatous condition, and has
been described in detail by Sigurdsson et al. (1957).

But the principal disease which engaged the attention of
Sigurdsson and his co-workers was rida (Icelandic: trembling)
now recognized as identical with scrapie (*la tremblante*; *Zittern-
krankheit*) of Western Europe. Scrapie has become a paradigm
amongst slow infections and a great deal of work has been ex-
pended on exploring its remarkable features. Whilst these diseases
were recognized as showing a well marked genetic influence and

occurred spontaneously, they could also be experimentally transmitted.

The characteristics of 'slow' infection tentatively set out by Sigurdsson (1954) were:

1. A very long interval period of latency to be reckoned in terms of months or even years rather than days or weeks.
2. A rather regular protracted course after clinical signs have appeared, usually eventuating in serious disease or death.
3. Limitation of the infection to a single host species with anatomical lesions in only a single organ or tissue system.

Whilst Sigurdsson recognized that these basic criteria might well need modification or amplification in the light of subsequent research, the enthusiasm with which his concept of 'slow' infection was received resulted in extension of the blanket title to many conditions for which the evidence was slender. By 1965 the list of conditions covered 3 quarto pages (Gajdusek et al. 1965) and it appeared that the label of 'slow infection' now vied with 'auto-immune disease' as embracing most conditions of obscure aetiology. Moreover, whilst Sigurdsson spoke of 'slow infections', others had begun to talk of slow 'viruses'. There is now evidence that viruses (e.g. measles) which ordinarily act in a well recognized acute manner may, under certain conditions, persist (or act *ab initio*) as agents capable of producing 'slow infections'. Furthermore, a clear distinction has not always been held between slow and latent or temperate infection, so that in the list of Gajdusek et al. (1965) rabies appears. Whilst rabies virus may certainly lie dormant in tissues for prolonged periods (perhaps for as long as 2 years), when it does produce disease it is of a fulminating kind quite different from Sigurdsson's conception. At this stage in our knowledge, 'slow infection' should be kept distinct in our thinking from latent infection.

Work on scrapie (the model of 'slow infections' still most widely studied) was much handicapped for many years by limitation of the disease, for all practical purposes, to sheep, in which the incubation extended from 18 months to 5 years. When, therefore, Chandler showed in 1961 that the disease might be established in mice with an 'incubation period' of some 5 to 8 months, he greatly facilitated its study. Later Chandler and Fisher (1963) went on to show it could also be established in rats, again with a much lesser incubation period (some 10 months). Bioassay extending over some 6 to 8 months has, until very recently, been the only method of demonstrating or titrating scrapie agent. Recently, however, Field and Shenton (1973a, 1974a) have evolved a method of establishing a diagnosis within 8 to 10 days on the basis of special lymphocyte sensitization as measured by the recently devised macrophage electrophoretic mobility (MEM) test (Field & Caspary 1970; Caspary & Field 1971). This will be considered further below.

Transmission attempts with human degenerative disease of the nervous system

Kuru, which in the local Fore dialect of the Eastern Central Highlands of New Guinea means 'to be afraid' or 'to tremble (with fear)', was brought to the attention of Western medicine by Gajdusek and Zigas (1957), though it seems to have been noted by European observers in the 1950s (Berndt 1954) or even the twenties (Williams 1923). Berndt regarded the disease as hysterical, describing patients who, 'walking with the aid of a stick or with the help of friends', showed 'involuntary twitchings' with 'lack of control over the limbs'. The disease appears to have been recognized by these Stone Age culture natives for some 40 to 50 years, though there are considerable difficulties in communication and time measurement (Alpers 1965). Early workers (e.g. Bennett et al. 1958, 1959) recorded that male kuru patients were born almost exclusively to kuru mothers, and postulated a genetic mechanism involving a single autosomal dominant gene. Fischer and Fischer (1960, 1963) were disinclined to accept a genetic basis for kuru, but thought some environmental factor must be at work.

Meanwhile Hadlow (1959) had drawn attention to the broad resemblance of the clinical and neuropathological features of human kuru and sheep scrapie. Whilst realizing that 'attempts to draw too close an analogy between diseases of man and lower animals are

attended by numerous pit-falls', Hadlow felt the resemblances were
sufficiently close to invite transmission attempts, and made the
seminal suggestion that 'it might be profitable . . . to examine the
possibility of the experimental induction of Kuru in a laboratory
primate', since 'the pathogenetic mechanisms involved in scrapie—
however unusual they may be—are unlikely to be unique in the
province of animal pathology'. An extensive programme of transmission experiments was accordingly undertaken at National
Institutes of Health, Bethesda (Gajdusek & Gibbs 1964) with a
large variety of animals and tissue cultures. Initially, success
attended only the inoculations made into chimpanzees, but since
then more readily available animals have been shown to be
susceptible and it seems probable that the widening of host range
ultimately to embrace tissue culture which occurred with poliomyelitis virus will take place also with the agents of 'slow infections'.

SCRAPIE

Animal range
Whilst the naturally occurring disease is one almost exclusively
of sheep, it has on rare occasions been reported in goats which
have been kept for prolonged periods in contact with scrapie-
affected sheep, either at pasture or indoors (Chelle 1942, kept
together from birth; Stamp 1962; Hourrigan et al. 1969; Dickinson et al. 1974; Buntain et al. 1974). In a sequential study of the
development of the special lymphocyte sensitization characteristic
of scrapie (see below) (Field & Shenton 1973, 1974b) in lambs
born of scrapie affected ewes, Shenton et al. (1975) found that the
special sensitivity established itself 18 months after the birth of
the lamb, before clinical signs supervened. Natural scrapie in
goats is likely to be a very rare event (Mackay & Smith 1961),
though the species may readily be infected by intracerebral
inoculation (Pattison et al. 1959). It also has been established in
mice (Chandler 1961) and in rats (Chandler & Fisher 1963).
Hamsters are susceptible (Zlotnik 1963) as also are gerbils, but
rabbits, by peripheral, intracerebral and oral routes, guinea pigs

and chimpanzees do not appear to be so. Crossing the species barrier is always attended by a prolonged incubation period (often with atypical pathology) which is reduced at subsequent passages. Mink encephalopathy is very probably scrapie established in this species through the feeding of infected meat (Burger & Hartshough 1965). It was first recognized in a few Wisconsin mink farms from about 1950 onwards. A severe epizootic in 1963 made it clear that a new entity was involved. The clinical and pathological features of the disease closely resemble scrapie—progressive central nervous disturbance with ingravescent locomotor incoordination (Burger & Hartshough 1965). Behavioural changes (failure of the animal to keep itself clean), excitability, anorexia, unsteadiness, hind quarter incoordination and occasionally convulsions occur. Later there is somnolence. There is a jerky stiff stepping gait, sometimes with a fine tremor. Vacuolation of grey matter is characteristic with neuronal vacuolation also.

The physical and chemical properties of the agent closely resemble those of scrapie. Passage in mink has an incubation period of 4 to 5 months (intracerebrally) or $6\frac{1}{2}$ to 8 months intramuscularly. The disease may well have been introduced by feeding infected meat. It has been passaged into albino ferrets, hamsters (Marsh et al. 1969), mice and rhesus monkey (Marsh et al. 1969) and squirrel monkeys (Eckroade et al. 1969).

Scrapie agent is present in all tissues of affected animals including afterbirth products (Pattison et al. 1972), so that spread under natural conditions has been suggested by these authors to occur through sheep eating voided fetal membranes at lambing time, or through lambs gulping amniotic fluid (Buntain et al. 1974). The high resistance of scrapie agent will, of course, contribute to pasture contamination by such membrane disintegration.

The problem of spread under natural conditions is a long-standing one in veterinary medicine, and as long ago as 1954 Sigurdsson recounted how all the sheep in the larger part of northern Iceland were destroyed in an attempt to eradicate maedi. This area included that in which rida had been prevalent. When healthy sheep were subsequently brought into these same areas once again, farmers were surprised to find that rida reappeared in the following years on the same farms in the recently introduced stock. Rida had not been known to occur in the areas from which the imported sheep had been taken, and it did not appear in the sheep from these same areas introduced onto farms which had previously been rida free. Sigurdsson was of the opinion that this constituted 'conclusive evidence that the virus of rida had survived outside the known host on the farms . . . and was ready to infect immediately the recently introduced sheep'. This Sigurdsson took as evidence that some intermediate host or vector might play a part in natural spread of the disease. Just how scrapie does in fact spread—assuming it is not under natural conditions an entirely genetically determined condition (Parry 1962, 1966)—is still not clear. In recent experiments, Brotherston et al. (1968) found that while at the Moredun Institute, Edinburgh, sheep and goats kept indoors for several years in direct contact with a succession of sheep affected by natural scrapie developed the disease, goats held in contact with experimentally induced scrapie in sheep (at the Animal Diseases Research Centre, A.R.C., Compton) failed to develop it. Clearly the difference might arise from differences in the natural and experimentally induced condition, or from vector presence (cf. Sigurdsson 1954).

Whilst the mechanism of natural transmission of scrapie remains in doubt, there is clear evidence of a genetic factor in the development of the condition (Parry 1962), so that different breeds show great variation in susceptibility to experimental infection (e.g. Herdwick 78%, Swaledale 54%, Dorset Down 0%; Gordon 1966). The interaction of exciting agent and genetic soil is of great importance in the development of slow infections.

Under experimental conditions the disease is commonly transmitted by intracerebral inoculation, though intramuscular, intraperitoneal or subcutaneous injection is successful after a somewhat prolonged incubation period. The disease is also readily transmitted to goats and sheep by the oral route (Pattison & Millson 1961), and in mice cannibalism is the probable manner in which it spreads from affected to normal mice within a cage (Pattison 1964). On the other hand the disease does not spread amongst mice by animal house fomites (sawdust, droppings, etc.) (Field &

Joyce 1970). There would appear to be a very transient 'viraemia' (even after intracerebral inoculation and after which blood is remarkably non-infective) (Field 1967b), and the segments of the neuraxis first affected (by astroglial hypertrophy—the first morphological response to scrapie agent) are those related to the injection site (Field 1967a). In this respect (but in few others) scrapie agent resembles a 'neurotropic virus'.

Association with multiple sclerosis

In 1965 Palsson et al. reported the emergence of scrapie in Icelandic sheep which had been injected intracerebrally with brain from the vicinity of an acute multiple sclerosis plaque with typical appearance (illustrated Field 1969). No independent confirmation of such a relation between multiple sclerosis and scrapie has appeared since these experiments, and recent immunological studies make it highly probable that the association is spurious and founded on some 'laboratory error' (Field et al. 1974) (see below).

Immunological tests

Scrapie Among the remarkable features accredited to scrapie infection is its failure to elicit immunological reaction. However, Gardner (1965) found that 'spleen preparations from scrapie-infected animals were much better from an antigenic point of view than were similar preparations from non-scrapie tissues', and suggested that 'some tissue components that are poorly antigenic in the non-scrapie spleen become improved antigenically in the scrapie spleen'. Gardner's experiments were limited to circulating antibody. With the development of a precise and consistent method of measuring lymphocyte sensitization (an important parameter of delayed hypersensitivity) to specific antigens, the study of scrapie and multiple sclerosis from this point of view was taken up. The method was devised primarily for the study of lymphocyte sensitization in multiple sclerosis and other neurological diseases and is called the macrophage electrophoretic mobility (MEM) test (Field & Caspary 1970, 1971; Caspary & Field 1971). In principle it depends upon the observation that when sensitized lymphocytes are brought into contact with specific antigen some lymphokine (MSF = macrophage slowing factor: which may be identical with the well recognized MIF) is liberated, with the property of causing normal guinea pig macrophages to travel more slowly in an electric field. Normal guinea pig macrophages may thus be used as an indicator system for the liberation of MSF and thus of lymphocyte recognition of antigen. The percentage slowing of the macrophages is a measure of their sensitization. An experimental protocol in extenso is given by Caspary and Field (1971).

Tissues from scrapie mice (or from similar mice injected with normal brain as controls) were inoculated into guinea pigs and some 8 days later the sensitization of the guinea pig lymphocyte to a suspension of scrapie and normal mouse brain was estimated. In other words, the ability of tissues from scrapie, as opposed to normal, mice to induce lymphocyte sensitization in guinea pigs was studied. It was found that reactivity of lymphocytes to scrapie brain was greater than to normal brain, even when the guinea pig had been injected with normal brain. However, this scrapie-normal difference (SND) was much greater when the guinea pig had been injected with scrapie tissue than with normal tissue. Such studies can be used for the diagnosis of scrapie in mice and indeed for its titration in the tissues (Field & Shenton 1972, 1973a, 1974a). Moreover, it has been found that the high SND induced in guinea pig lymphocytes with scrapie tissues only begins to be associated with scrapie injected mouse brain 50 days after intracerebral inoculation (at a time when the earliest morphological changes (astroglial hypertrophy) are not yet present). Other nonneural tissues, e.g. spleen, also induce the same high SND on the part of the lymphocytes of an injected guinea pig (Field & Shenton 1973). The method has also been used to trace the presence of scrapie agent activity in neuronal and glial compartments of scrapie mouse brain. Contrary to what had been expected, titre was higher in the neuronal than in the glial compartment (Narang et al. 1972). Further experiments have shown that mouse brain in which astroglial hypertrophy had been induced by cuprizone feeding (Pattison & Jebbett 1971) produced the same high SND in guinea pig lymphocytes. Indeed, when kuru or Jakob–Creutzfeldt brain material was injected into guinea pigs, the same high SND was induced in their lymphocytes. It would, therefore, appear that the high SND is associated rather with subtle membrane changes which, in the case of the brain but not in other tissues, are manifested by astrogliosis (Field & Shenton 1973e).

When lymphocytes from sheep affected with natural scrapie are separated from blood and tested for reactivity against scrapie and normal mouse brain suspensions, the SND is considerably greater than it is with lymphocytes from normal sheep. Other neurological diseases of sheep (e.g. Border disease) do not show high SND, so that the method can be used for the diagnosis of natural scrapie in the sheep (Field & Shenton 1973).

Multiple sclerosis Whilst the aetiology of multiple sclerosis remains unknown, it is difficult to exclude participation of some immunological mechanism in the evolution of the clinical picture, especially during recurrent episodes of illness. However, the existence of a group of diseases with very prolonged incubation period has led to revival of interest in an infective aetiology—with an agent producing a slow type of infection. The link with scrapie suggested by Palsson et al. (1965) has been described above, but recent developments make it probable that it was an error.

Lymphocytes from the blood of patients with multiple sclerosis show well marked sensitization to encephalitogenic factor (EF) (Caspary & Field 1965), but this is also found in all diseases (including traumatic) which involve parenchymatous destruction of nervous tissue (Caspary & Field 1970), so that there is nothing specific to multiple sclerosis in this respect. However, there have been suggestions that multiple sclerosis may develop against a background of abnormal handling of unsaturated fatty acids (Thompson 1966), and recently it has been suggested (Turnell et al. 1973) that corticosteroids may act through influencing the level of free fatty acids. In multiple sclerosis, too, it has long been claimed that the brain (even in apparently unaffected areas) is deficient in unsaturated fatty acids (Baker et al. 1963) and a decrease in linoleate has been recorded in serum (Baker et al. 1965). Recently, Millar et al. (1973) have reported a beneficial effect of administration of sunflower seed oil (linoleic acid) to patients with multiple sclerosis, at least in diminishing the number and severity of attacks over a period of 2 years.

The suggestion that linoleic acid might dampen down the ability of lymphocytes to interact with antigen, coupled with the beneficial effect of linoleic acid in multiple sclerosis, led to the theoretical possibility that lymphocytes in multiple sclerosis might be specially sensitive to linoleic acid. The prophylactic effect of exhibition of LA might thus be due to prevention of lymphocyte recognition of putative antigen (EF) in situ in myelin. Direct experiment confirmed these theoretical ideas. It was found that lymphocytes from multiple sclerosis patients were indeed more sensitive to linoleic acid than were those from either normal subjects or those affected with other neurological diseases. Response of lymphocytes to EF could not be tested in normal subjects (where it is always very low), but suppression of lymphocyte recognition of EF in multiple sclerosis with linoleic acid was much greater than in other neurological diseases (87·9% as against 45·2%). Moreover, the same increased susceptibility of multiple sclerosis cells to linoleic acid was shown when other antigens such as F1 thyroid (thyroglobulin, towards which there is universal sensitization) or PPD was studied. With F1 thyroid multiple sclerosis cells gave a reduction of 90·1% response when linoleic acid was incorporated in the in vitro test system; other neurological diseases gave 46·4%, whilst normal lymphocytes gave 54·7% (Mertin et al. 1973). A more extended series of results has also been published (Field et al. 1974) indicating that the degree of suppressive activity of linoleic acid on lymphocytic interaction with antigen (F1 of thyroid is commonly used) is specifically increased in multiple sclerosis. Restriction of the results is so close that they may be used as a specific in vitro test for the disease.

Transmission experiments

RELATION OF MULTIPLE SCLEROSIS TO SCRAPIE

In 1947 Campbell et al. reported the development of multiple sclerosis in 4 of 7 research workers at Cambridge studying sway-back in sheep. Whilst it is now known that swayback is almost certainly a dysmyelogenesis in lambs associated with copper (and perhaps other trace element) deficiency in the pasture on which ewes are raised, Campbell's cases were striking and their attribution to chance seemed very remote. Sutherland and Wilson (1951) were unsuccessful in their attempts to transmit the disease to sheep by injection of blood and spinal fluid from multiple sclerosis cases, although they observed their animals over a period of 17 months. However, the existence of 'slow' infections made clear by Sigurdsson (1954) stimulated further examination of the possibility that multiple sclerosis might be of this nature (probably supplemented by some immunological mechanism which would more readily account for dramatically sudden clinical bouts). Indeed, the epidemiological data of multiple sclerosis could be so arranged (Schapira et al. 1963) as to appear to support some exogenous causal agency with a long pre-clinical incubation period.

In 1965 Palsson et al. reported the highly unexpected emergence of scrapie in Icelandic sheep after intracerebral inoculation with material from an acute multiple sclerosis plaque. On second passage, the incubation period was reduced from 18·5 months to 10·8 months (a phenomenon expected when the species barrier is crossed; but also to be expected if the inoculum were lightly contaminated with scrapie or disease was being 'lit up' in sheep). Repetition with the original material gave 2 of 5 sheep positive with the original long incubation period. At the time of these experiments, scrapie was not being worked with in Newcastle.

Attempts to repeat the Icelandic experiments (both at Newcastle and A.R.C. Compton, Mr T. H. Pattison) were unsuccessful, as they were, too, in Northern Ireland (Dick et al. 1965). Moreover, material sent by Campbell et al. (1963) from a case of subacute encephalitis associated with necrotizing myelitis was also briefly reported as producing a scrapie-like condition in Icelandic sheep, so that Dick et al. (1965) suggested there may have been an activation of latent rida by the inoculation of the diseased brain material (though not from the normal control material).

In 1966 Field reported production of scrapie in mice after blind passage of multiple sclerosis biopsy material and X-irradiation. Unfortunately, scrapie had already been imported into the Unit (following the Icelandic findings) and, as the author himself wrote, it is 'important that attempts to pass multiple sclerosis into mice should be made in laboratories not working with scrapie material at all'. In later attempts it proved impossible to transmit disease to mice.

Whilst these reports stimulated much interest in scrapie and the nature of the agent, it is now most likely that they were based upon some 'laboratory error', as will appear below.

With the development of an in vitro test for multiple sclerosis, sheep suffering from natural scrapie were tested as compared with normal sheep. They were found not to show the increased lymphocyte susceptibility to suppression of linoleic acid characteristic of multiple sclerosis (Field et al. 1974), and the association of multiple sclerosis and scrapie is correspondingly weakened. Added to this is the observation that in chimpanzees injected with multiple sclerosis brain material (the same as produced scrapie in the Icelandic sheep reported by Palsson et al. 1965) an exaggerated SND was not found when the lymphocytes were tested with scrapie and normal mouse brain antigens, though it did develop after kuru or Jakob-Creutzfeldt brain had been injected into chimpanzees (Field & Shenton 1974b). This again suggests that multiple sclerosis behaves differently from recognized 'slow' infections, and the writer now feels that the observation in 1965 and the Newcastle finding in 1966 must rest upon some laboratory error. However, those reports were fertile in the sense that they directed much attention to the viral aspects of multiple sclerosis. Currently the mantle seems to have fallen upon measles (see below).

KURU

Kuru was the first human disease to be shown due to 'slow' infection. The disease itself has declined sharply in incidence from 220 cases registered in 1959 to 126 in 1966 and 86 in 1970, the decline being greater amongst women and children, so that no cases in children under 12 have been found in the last few years. In 1974 there are probably no more than 30 to 40 cases left. Circumstantial evidence suggests the spread of kuru is associated with the practice of cannibalism, which has certainly declined abruptly since about 1957. Probably the excess of cases amongst women and children is associated with ingestion of brain and spleen— more highly infectious than muscle—though (since it is now clear that peripheral inoculation may produce the disease in animals) infection through cuts, nose-picking or through the conjunctiva may have occurred. It is possible that some genetic 'soil' may be necessary for the development of the disease. A kuru-like condition has been described in Europe (Schaltenbrand et al. 1968), but no case has ever occurred amongst the Caucasians who have been in contact with kuru patients, so that infectivity under ordinary conditions is certainly very low (see below).

The original transmission of human kuru to chimpanzees was carried out in Washington by Gajdusek (1966). Up to 1973, primary transmission has been from 11 human brains into 19 animals, with incubation periods of 14 to 39 months. In subsequent passages, the incubation period (as is, in general, the case when the species barrier is crossed) dropped markedly to 10 to 18 months (mean: 22 to 11 months). In Newcastle, intramuscular injection of 1 ml of 10 : 1 suspension of cerebral cortex together with white matter of a second passage kuru chimpanzee (kindly supplied by Dr D. C. Gajdusek) has produced clinical disease in 18 months in 2 animals. Whilst Gajdusek and co-workers have emphasized the considerable similarity in clinical features between kuru in man and chimpanzee, this has not been specially striking in Newcastle. In these animals, a fine tremor preceded incoordination by 2 or 3 months and trunkal ataxia was never marked, though the

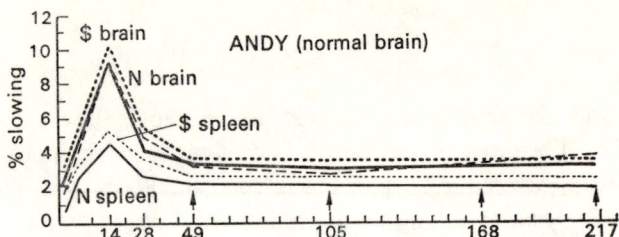

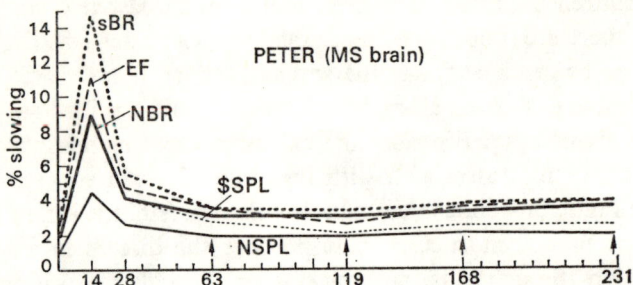

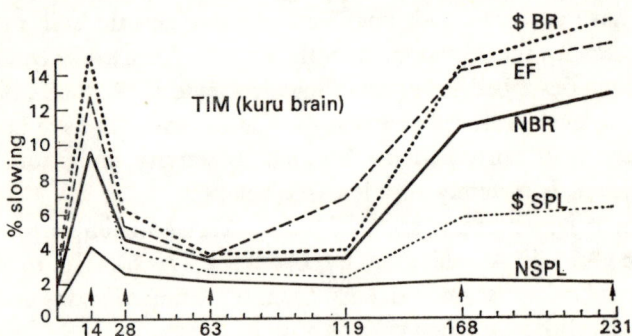

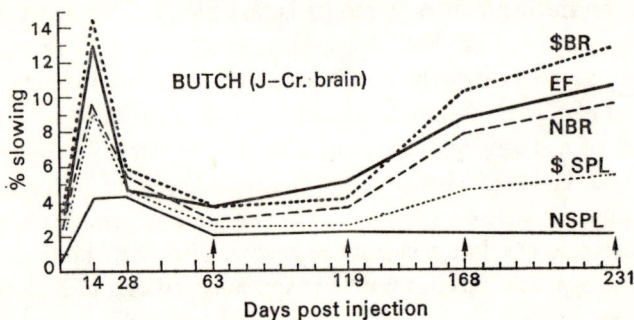

Fig. 8. Lymphocytes removed from chimpanzee at intervals shown and tested for sensitization against normal brain, scrapie brain (both of mouse), normal and scrapie spleen (mouse) and encephalitogenic factor (EF) made from human brain. S=scrapie.

a, Andy. Normal brain injected into chimpanzee. Note the initial response in which SND (scrapie normal difference) is small on testing with either brain or spleen. There is no later secondary response as occurs when kuru or Jakob–Creutzfeldt disease establishes itself.

b, Peter. Multiple sclerosis brain injected into chimpanzee (the same multiple sclerosis material as that from which scrapie emerged in Iceland). Note the initial response in which there is a large SND for both brain and spleen antigens. There is also a considerable EF response. There is no secondary response because no infection of slow type has established itself. The large initial SND is seen also in guinea pigs injected with multiple sclerosis brain.

c, Tim. Kuru brain injected into chimpanzee. Note the initial response in which there is a high SND for both brain and spleen as well as an EF response (since destroyed brain was injected). Note the secondary rise in EF response after 63 days—indicative of new brain destruction with auto-sensitization. Note the secondary rise in sensitization to normal and scrapie brain with high SND as infection becomes established. The animals were yet clinically normal. Note that the EF response occurs before the special scrapie response, suggesting that brain destruction has preceded the glial response.

d, Butch. Jakob–Creutzfeldt brain injected into chimpanzee. Note same phenomena as with Tim.

In the case of Tim and Butch, i.e. injection of kuru or Jakob–Creuzfeldt material, infection has established itself with immunological changes. This has not been so with the multiple sclerosis brain injection.

animals were readily pushed over and seemed insecure in estimating a jump distance so that they were reluctant to undertake it.

Histologically, changes were similar in both animals. Minute vacuolation was widespread throughout the grey matter and not especially marked in the spinal cord, despite the inoculation into the limbs. Detailed description of the histology has been published by Beck et al. (1966).

In a second Newcastle experiment 4 chimpanzees were injected: one with normal brain suspension (1·0 ml of 10% intramuscularly); one with the original brain (Sell) which had apparently produced scrapie in Icelandic sheep; one with brain from a well-developed case of Jakob–Creutzfeldt disease; and one with kuru. The 4 animals were allowed to mix freely, an important objective of the experiment being to find out if, under these conditions, either the control (injected with normal brain) or the animal injected with multiple sclerosis brain (shown by Gajdusek and co-workers to produce no disease) would contract either Jakob–Creutzfeldt disease or kuru. Since it is probable that these two diseases are identical, and Jakob–Creutzfeldt disease is currently nursed in open neurological wards, infectivity was being tested under ordinary conditions. Unfortunately, the main objective of the experiment was defeated by action of the Medical Research Council, but important immunological observations were made before this occurred. Lymphocyte sensitization to EF and to scrapie and normal brain was determined in each animal before inoculation and at intervals afterwards (Fig. 8). It can be seen that, whilst the injection of multiple sclerosis, kuru or Jakob–Creutzfeldt brain leads to a temporary rise in sensitization to EF and high SND, these are restored to baseline by 28 days. This immediate response appears associated with the astrogliosis in these brains (Field & Shenton 1973). No immediate response is shown by the animal inoculated with normal brain. At 119 days sensitization to EF began to rise above baseline in the case of the animals injected with kuru and Jakob–Creutzfeldt disease material but not in those inoculated with normal or multiple sclerosis brain, indicating brain destruction to which there has been secondary sensitization (Caspary & Field 1970). By 168 days EF sensitization has increased markedly in these 2 animals, though the normal and multiple sclerosis animals' EF sensitization remained at baseline, indicating no parenchymatous destruction. At this point, however, i.e. later than the earliest EF change, lymphocyte reactivity to scrapie brain (and spleen) had clearly outstripped that to the corresponding normal tissues so that the SND was elevated (Fig. 9) in the case of the kuru and Jakob–Creutzfeldt animals. Disease has established itself in these latter animals but not in the former two. A fuller interpretation has been considered elsewhere (Field & Shenton 1973), but here the important point is that, whilst the kuru and Jakob–Creutzfeldt inoculations have 'taken', the multiple sclerosis one has not. Unfortunately, for reasons beyond the writer's control, it was not possible to adhere to the original plan and keep the unaffected animals for much longer periods.

Failure of evidence of the establishment of any slowly progressive change in the brain (one of Sigurdsson's primary

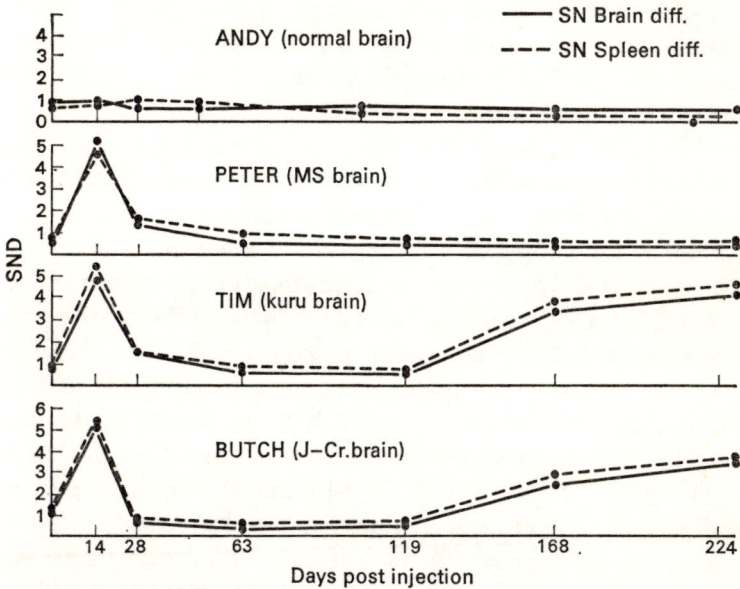

Fig. 9. Scrapie normal difference in degree of lymphocyte sensitization shown for both brain and spleen at intervals after the original injection. Animals as in Fig. 8.

Note no initial peak of SND in Andy (injected with normal brain). The initial peak in Peter injected with multiple sclerosis brain is characteristic. The secondary peaks denote the establishment of infection.

All measurements of lymphocyte sensitization throughout these experiments were carried out by Mr B. K. Shenton.

characteristics of 'slow' infections), coupled with the failure of scrapie sheep to give a positive multiple sclerosis test, combine to make very unlikely the association of scrapie with multiple sclerosis suggested by the 1965 and 1966 reports described above.

The development of sensitization to EF before a 'high' SND which appears to be dependent upon astroglial reaction (Field &

Shenton 1973) suggests that the agent of kuru and Jakob–Creutz-feldt disease causes damage to neural elements first and that the astroglial reaction is a secondary phenomenon, as is commonly the case in neuropathological changes. All who have worked on the histology of scrapie are, however, unanimous in emphasizing astroglial hypertrophy as the earliest recognizable morphological change, and this seems to be true of kuru and Jakob–Creutzfeldt disease also. Clearly, however, subtle degenerative or biochemical changes in nervous elements may suffice to set in train sensitization to EF before morphological changes are recognizable in the microscope. That scrapie agent, despite the earliest histological changes, may proliferate in neurones rather than in glia is supported by the finding of a higher titre of agent in the neuronal than in the glial compartment of brain in early cases in the mouse.

Apart from chimpanzees, kuru has now also been passaged directly from human brain into 3 species of South American monkeys, the spider (*Ateles geoffreyi*), the capuchin (*Cebes apella*) and the squirrel (*Saimizi sciureus*) with an incubation period ranging from 20 to 51 months (average 30 months) (Gajdusek et al. 1968). Second passage in capuchins has again caused a marked reduction in incubation period (9 to 12 months). Clearly it is more practicable to work with these South American monkeys, though they are far more demanding in temperature and humidity conditions and less hardy than chimpanzees. Recently it has been claimed that kuru has been passed into 1 of 4 Rhesus monkeys (*Macaca mulatta*) $8\frac{1}{2}$ years after inoculation intracerebrally and intravenously with a 10% suspension of brain tissue from a human kuru patient (Gajdusek & Gibbs 1972).

JAKOB–CREUTZFELDT DISEASE
(SUBACUTE SPONGIFORM ENCEPHALOPATHY)

Whilst this disease is for the most part sporadic, a genetic element undoubtedly exists, as exemplified in the remarkable Backer family, in which 14 cases, spread over 4 generations, appear to be associated with a single dominant gene; family B (Friede & De Jong 1964) in which a father and 3 daughters were affected; and the family R (Davison & Rabiner 1940) in which 2 brothers and 1 sister were affected (though because of the association with amyotrophic lateral sclerosis and the rather younger age of onset, some neurologists—though not Kirschbaum (1968)—would exclude these). Another familial example involving a grandmother, a mother and a son, with 2 maternal aunts succumbing to a rapidly dementing disease, was reported by Bonduelle et al. (1971). Jellinger and Seitelberger (1972) have reported a conjugal example.

The resemblance of Jakob–Creutzfeldt disease to kuru was appreciated early by Klatzo et al. (1959) who, in attempting to fit kuru into the context of known pathological entities, concluded that it was with 'Creutzfeldt–Jacob (*sic*) disease . . . (that kuru) . . . appears to be closest in resemblance'. Indeed efforts to demonstrate an infective aetiology of Jakob–Creutzfeldt disease were based entirely on the striking similarity in the neuropathological lesions, the differences being mainly in distribution and intensity. In a recent EEG study of chimpanzees inoculated with kuru or Jakob–Creutzfeldt material, changes in the former were found to be only mild whereas the latter animals showed severe EEG changes which, however, lacked the typical spike sequence seen in human patients (Niedermeyer et al. 1972).

The disease has been transmitted to chimpanzees by the Washington workers Gibbs et al. (1968) who recorded that, while the changes in the brain had certain features in common with kuru, 'there were other features not characteristic of kuru that enabled this brain to be easily distinguished from that of the animal with experimental kuru'. However, subsequent studies (as has been the case with the Newcastle kuru and Jakob–Creutzfeldt material) have tended to diminish the emphasis on these differences. Indeed Field (1969), in reviewing slow infections of the nervous system, thought it 'highly probable that . . . (Jakob–Creutzfeldt disease) . . . will turn out to be kuru–scrapie', and it is likely that Jakob–Creutzfeldt disease is the Western analogue of kuru. Gibbs and Gajdusek (1971) have speculated that 'the initial source of kuru agent might have been a rare sporadic occurence of a case of Jakob–Creutzfeldt disease in a Fore New Guinea Highlander, and that the widespread contamination of the people in the mourning ritual of cannibalistic consumption of dead relatives, with inoculation of themselves and their infants, may have only served to disperse the infection widely in a pseudo-genetic pattern determined by the familial pattern of mourning for kinsmen who were kuru victims.'

Like kuru, Jakob–Creutzfeldt disease has also been transmitted to New World (spider) monkeys (Gajdusek & Gibbs 1971) from 13 cases of human disease. In chimpanzees intracerebral inoculation gave an incubation period of 11 to 16 months. (The Newcastle case had an incubation period of 14 months to the beginning of signs.) Subsequent passage has maintained the same incubation period. It has also been transmitted to the three South American monkeys mentioned above, as well as the woolly monkey (*Lago-thrix lagothrica*). The incubation periods were slightly different—23 to 29 months (Gajdusek & Gibbs 1973).

TISSUE CULTURE

Clearly, as time goes by, it is becoming possible to use more readily available animals for experimental work on scrapie, kuru and Jakob–Creutzfeldt disease. There seems no reason why, like poliomyelitis virus, the agent of these diseases should not be ultimately kept in tissue culture. Gustaffson and Kanitz (1965) and Field and Windsor (1966) reported that explants of scrapie-affected mouse brain grew with greater vigour than those from similarly aged normal brain. This has been confirmed by others (Haig & Pattison 1967) and it is now known that infective scrapie agents can replicate (to low titre) for more than one hundred subcultures (Haig & Clarke 1971). There would appear to be much scope for explanation experiments of this type, and it would be of great interest to determine whether the rapid immunological titration method of Field and Shenton (1973) might be applied to cultures, so that estimations would be very greatly expedited.

Both kuru and Jakob–Creutzfeldt infectivity persist in explanted human and animal brain tissue (Gajdusek et al. 1972) since inocula prepared from such explants have produced characteristic disease in chimpanzees. Kuru has been found to persist for at least 77 days, and Jakob–Creutzfeldt for at least 255 days. The type of cell which maintains the agent cannot be certainly ascertained because the clear astroglial type of cell seen in an early explant soon becomes converted into a flattened macrophage-like cell or more spindle-like cells which resemble fibroblasts, so that morphology is of little value in predicating a cell type which has been maintained in culture for some time. Significantly, the cells in which the agent undergoes low level replication do not show pathological change. The same is true of scrapie.

There is no evidence of interferon production in tissue cultures of kuru or Jakob–Creutzfeldt brain, and indeed interferon is not produced in mice affected by scrapie (Gresser & Pattison 1968), nor does it appear to influence the course of the disease (Field et al. 1969). Interferon appears without effect upon the development of Jakob–Creutzfeldt disease in chimpanzees (Gajdusek & Gibbs 1973).

An interesting collateral finding from prolonged maintenance of tissue culture explants of chimpanzee brain has been the emergence of a host of 'latent' viruses (Basnight et al. 1970: Gajdusek et al. 1972). C-type particles have been seen in the Jakob–Creutzfeldt chimpanzee brain in Newcastle, but none of these is likely to be significant for the development of disease.

RELATION OF SLOW INFECTION TO THE AGEING PROCESS

Field (1967c) pointed out some of the resemblances between the changes found in the young animal with scrapie and those encountered normally in old age (e.g. astroglial hypertrophy, amyloid bodies, orientated tubules within axis cylinders, etc.). Amyloid plaques are said to occur in about 60% of patients with kuru (including children) (Gajdusek & Gibbs 1973), and they are also present in Jakob–Creutzfeldt disease. Recently it has been found that srapie-like antigenic determinants appear in normal tissues as they age. Indeed, an immunological ageing chart may be constructed (Field & Shenton 1973a). These changes are found both in man and mouse. They can be detected by injecting tissues from an animal of known age into a guinea pig and measuring the degree to which the guinea pig's lymphocytes become sensitized to scrapie brain (or spleen) some 8 days later. Thymectomy (in the neonatal mouse) greatly accelerates the development of scrapie-like antigens in tissues (Field & Shenton 1973b) and this may be held up by implants of thymus (Field & Shenton 1973c). The exact relation of the scrapie-like antigen making its appearance progressively with age to that actually present in tissues of mice or sheep suffering from scrapie is not yet determined, though it should be amenable to the combination of affinity column chromatography and the MEM test in the manner in which it has been used for studying the relation between EF and measles antigens (McDermott et al. 1974) (see below).

It has been suggested that some of the changes in the ageing brain may result from activation of latent viruses with ageing (Gajdusek 1971). However, the author's view is that ageing changes in tissues are associated with physicochemical alterations in cellular membranes resulting in the appearance of antigenic determinants which also make their appearance in the tissues of young scrapie animals. Whether scrapie is due to an 'agent' or represents a self-inducing change in tissues (Field 1967c) remains to be determined. Certainly prolonged search has not led to the recognition of any particular agent in tissues (cf. Narang & Field 1973). For the author, the presence of various viruses in ageing tissue may well represent their emergence from a latent state when the milieu becomes less satisfactory (ageing), rather than a causal relationship with the changes of ageing.

THE PROBLEM OF MEASLES

Encephalitis as a sequel to clinical measles has long been recognized and is responsive in most cases to ACTH with a *restitutio ad integrum.* Such incidents have no established relationship to multiple sclerosis, though they might, of course, signify the occasion on which measles virus reaches the central nervous system.

The association of measles and multiple sclerosis stems from the original report by Adams and Imagawa (1962) that (on the average) the titre of measles antibody was higher in a group of multiple sclerosis patients than in normals. Numerous studies followed, for the most part without other neurological diseases as controls as well as normal subjects. It cannot be too strongly emphasized that, in order that a phenomenon may be established as characteristic of multiple sclerosis, other neurological diseases must also be examined. Amongst these, it is only those with well marked parenchymatous destruction of nervous tissue which are valid controls, since clearly comparison of multiple sclerosis with migraine or cryptogenic epilepsy is not adequate. And amongst other neurological diseases, neurosyphilis is perhaps the best control condition, since here, too, there is extensive nervous tissue destruction, very well marked lymphocyte sensitization to EF (indeed commonly greater in degree than in multiple sclerosis itself; Caspary & Field 1974), and gamma globulin level is elevated in spinal fluid.

Whilst the notion of multiple sclerosis as being in some way associated with measles, either as a persistent infection following clinical measles or as a 'slow' infection *ab initio*, has been much encouraged by recent developments in the elucidation of subacute sclerosing panencephalitis (SSPE), there are several very important differences. Whatever the method used for measurement, the titres reported in multiple sclerosis are not high in comparison with SSPE and must be assessed in the light of the study by Berman et al. (1968) of the persistence of haemagglutinating anti-measles antibody titre in children over seven years after natural measles attacks. This shows occasional persistence of quite high titres comparable with those seen in multiple sclerosis patients. In addition, there have been reports which have failed to confirm high measles titres (Ross et al. 1965: Just et al. 1967). Skin sensitivity, too, is not increased (Sever & Kurtzke 1969), whilst

Henson et al. (1970) have found titres as high in healthy siblings as in multiple sclerosis sufferers (with female siblings on the whole higher than males). Whilst few of the numerous results reported (recently summarized by McAlpine et al. 1973) reach a significance of $P < 0.01$, Caspary et al. (1969) have pointed out that the P value depends upon the manner in which the data are analysed. Very high measles and rubella antibody titres have also been found associated with hepatitis, systemic lupus erythematosus and infectious mononucleosis (Laitinen & Vaheri 1974).

Recently, using the MEM test for lymphocyte sensitization, no difference has been found in cellular sensitization to measles antigen in multiple sclerosis as compared with normal subjects (unpublished).

However, despite these findings, the idea that measles is concerned in the aetiology of multiple sclerosis persists. Electron-microscopic observations of dubious significance (since similar 'measles' tubules have been reported in material from patients with lupus erythematosus) (Norton 1969; Prineas 1972; Klippel et al. 1973; Narang & Field 1973). Isolation of measles from a brain biopsy of multiple sclerosis (Field et al. 1973) has been reported though the authors treat this with great caution since measles was being worked with in the laboratory. Ter Meulen et al. (1972) have recorded the emergence of nucleocapsids and virions of para-influenza type in cultures of brain cells from cases of multiple sclerosis. This important work awaits expansion. Finnish and Swedish workers (Salmi et al. 1972) emphasize that antibodies to different components of the measles virion are detectable in multiple sclerosis serum. By using a combination of affinity chromatography and cell-titration with the MEM method (measuring the macrophage response given by decreasing numbers of lymphocytes), McDermott et al. (1974) have shown that measles virus shares antigenic determinants with EF. Thus, when measles antigen is put into a Bio-Gel column, it is able to filter out a considerable number of lymphocytes which are sensitized to EF and vice versa. Neutral materials such as mumps antigen have no effect. Lymphocytes from patients with other neurological diseases show the same effects, since they, too, are sensitized to EF. Of special interest would be such a study with lymphocytes from patients with neurosyphilis. The crucial experiments with measles virus fractions and EF have not been done (Field 1973). However, the sharing of antigenic determinants between EF and measles virus would appear to be adequate to account for the titres observed in circulating antibody studies. The relation between measles and EF antigens has been further followed both in the natural disease and in injected animals (Field et al. 1973) and the possible significance of this antigenic sharing pathogenesis of multiple sclerosis elaborated (Field 1973). Indeed the experimental results which demonstrate increased lymphocyte sensitization to EF after inoculation of common viral agents other than measles suggest that several may contribute to the development of the disease. In addition, the author has seen four children who were under the age of ten at onset of what, on the basis of the MEM test (Field et al. 1974a), would be diagnosed as multiple sclerosis. In all lymphocytic response against measles was diminished. Much remains to be explored in this field, but it seems possible that there is a group of childhood cases of multiple sclerosis associated with defective defence against measles allowing of the establishment of the agent as a 'slow' infection. To this, of course, auto-aggressive changes might be superadded. The measles agent might well be in a defective form.

Clearly the relation of measles to multiple sclerosis is much less securely established than it is in SSPE and it seems possible that the genetic background may be of determining importance in the evolution of multiple sclerosis. The familial background of the disease is well recognized (Mackay & Myrcanthopoulos 1966) and has recently been further explored by Field et al. (1974) with the MEM test. There would appear to be an inborn increased sensitivity of lymphocyte to suppression by linoleic acid in multiple sclerosis and the possible effect this might have on the ability of measles to establish itself in the nervous system, especially after a clinical attack of the disease, remains to be explored (see above).

MISCELLANEOUS 'SLOW' INFECTIONS OF THE
CENTRAL NERVOUS SYSTEM

*Subacute sclerosing panencephalitis (SSPE; van Bogaert;
Dawson's inclusion body encephalitis)*

This very rare disease (about one in a million) is now reasonably
securely associated with measles virus. The presence of tubular
structures similar to the nucleocapsids of the measles–distemper
group of paramyxoviruses within the intranuclear inclusions found
in the disease first drew attention to measles, and the association
was much strengthened by Connolly et al.'s (1967) demonstration
of measles viral antigen within brain cells of patients with SSPE.
Unusually high measles antibody titres have been reported by
many authors, especially with progression of the illness (Horta-
Barbosa et al. 1970) and also in brain homogenates (ter Meulen
et al. 1969). Brain cell cultures have led to the isolation of measles
virus (reviewed by Thormar 1971). The SSPE strains isolated
from different patients have, however, shown some different
characteristics in culture growths and, in general, have been more
neurotropic in laboratory animals than are wild measles strains
(Byington et al. 1970; Lehrich et al. 1970; Payne 1971), causing
an acute encephalitis in suckling hamsters fatal in 1 to 2 days.
This is a doubtful transmission, even though the virus can easily
be recovered from the baby hamster brain. Périer et al. (1968)
observed encephalitis in cynomologus monkeys 12 to 18 days after
intracerebral inoculation of human material. Other monkeys
developed some evidence of neurological disease 7 to 15 months
after inoculation, but later recovered, and at autopsy no changes
were seen. Katz et al. (1968, 1970) injected 10% suspensions of
brain tissue from human SSPE patients into young adult ferrets
and produced a neurological disease with ataxia, loss of interest in
the environment and some posterior spasticity some five months
later. None developed measles antibodies. Autopsy revealed
gliosis, perivascular cuffing and neuronophagia. Disease was produced (with a shortened incubation period of three months) by
passage. EEG changes characteristic of SSPE have not been

observed in ferrets (Niedermeyer et al. 1972). Tissue culture suspensions of SSPE brain explants (Katz et al. 1970) also produced encephalitis in ferrets, but with the very short incubation period of two weeks. The failure to isolate measles virus in these experiments suggests that, if this agent is implicated, it may well be in a defective form. Johnson (1970) has discussed 3 possibilities: (*a*) an abnormal host response to measles virus infection; (*b*) an unusual measles virus causing 'slow' infection in an otherwise normal host; and (*c*) interaction of measles with a second agent. This last suggestion has been elaborated by Horta-Barbosa et al. (1970) and by ter Meulen et al. (1970). It is possible that a papovavirus is the collaborator (Barbanti-Brodano et al. 1970; Koprowski et al. 1970).

Kim et al. (1970) have observed the development of an SSPE like disease in the baboon, but no virus has been cultivated.

Progressive multifocal leucencephalopathy (PML)
This rare condition most commonly accompanies lymphoproliferative conditions (such as Hodgkin's disease), cancers or sarcoidosis, especially when immunosuppressive therapy has been instituted. The pathological changes are primarily multiple foci of demyelination surrounded by enlarged abnormal oligodendrocytes and (later) giant astrocytes with intranuclear inclusions. In the electron microscope the nuclei of oligodendrocytes contain large numbers of a papovavirus particle (possibly SV 40) (Zu Rhein 1969a, b). Despite their strikingly consistent occurrence, there is no evidence that they are destructive and their exact role is unknown. It seems probable that the papovavirus lies dormant and becomes a fully formed recognizable virion under conditions of immunosuppression or malignant disease.

No comparable disease appears to have been induced in animals.

Epilepsia partialis continua (Kojewnikoff's syndrome)
This disease, which is very rare in this country, has been thought to be due to a chronic focal encephalitis tick borne in origin in the Soviet Union (Russian spring–summer encephalitis virus) (Asher 1971). No transfer experiments have been reported.

Visna

This disease of sheep has only marginal interest for human neuropathologists. Hailed at first as a 'demyelinating disease' of sheep occurring spontaneously in Iceland, it is now known to be a chronic granulomatous periventricular or juxtaventricular degeneration in the course of which myelin (along with other parenchymatous elements) is destroyed. The disease has considerable theoretical interest, since the causal virus, which is clearly defined in the electron microscope (e.g. Coward et al. 1970), is closely related to that of maedi (a 'slow' pneumonitis). Indeed it seems highly probable that visna and maedi agents are strains of the same virus (Thormar 1971). Clinically, cases of visna were first observed in Iceland between 1935 and 1940 as sporadic nervous disease in flocks where maedi was widespread. Visna has been thoroughly studied in Iceland (Thormar 1967; Thormar & Palsson 1967) and the virus found in spina fluid, blood and saliva of infected sheep during the long preclinical period. The virus may be present in brain or lungs for years before changes occur. Curiously, complement fixing antibodies are formed in this disease.

The virus has been grown in cell cultures from sheep and cattle, but not from small laboratory animals (Harter et al. 1968; Harter 1969). The experimental animal remains the sheep.

Following the study of visna in Iceland, the progressive lung indurations which had been recognized in other countries have been compared with visna–maedi. Some serological relationships with zwegerziekte in Holland and progressive pneumonia of sheep in Montana, USA, have been established. A review of these fascinating relationships has recently been made by Thormar (1971). A visna-like encephalitis has been described in Dutch flocks with the lung disease (Ressang et al. 1966). However, a curious feature is the great variation in the neurological manifestations of visna–maedi infection in different countries. In Iceland visna was very common in a restricted area, whilst elsewhere it has remained rare. Clearly much remains to study of the interaction of agent and genetic soil in the evolution of all 'slow' infections, and for this visna is an excellent model.

CONCLUSIONS

The seminal work of Sigurdsson and his school introduced a new concept into our ideas of 'infection'—that the 'incubation period' might last one-quarter or even one-third of an animal's life. Application of this new idea has established the transmissibility of human kuru and Jakob–Creutzfeldt disease. Alzheimer's disease (pre-senile dementia) seems likely to be another. So far multiple sclerosis has not been transmitted and reports of its connection with scrapie are almost certainly based upon laboratory error. However, this has proved fertile in directing considerable attention to exploring the possibility that multiple sclerosis may be of the nature of a 'slow' infection, perhaps even by a banal virus (for which the principal contemporary candidate is measles). Measles appears to be in some way involved (perhaps in association with another helper virus) in SSPE.

The study of animal diseases, especially scrapie and visna, have warned of the peculiarities which may be encountered in the nature and properties of the agents possibly concerned in human disease.

The oft-repeated statement that 'slow' infections are not associated with immunological changes is clearly not true for visna–maedi and has recently been shown to require modification in scrapie, kuru and Jakob–Creutzfeldt disease. Despite intensive search, a convincing virus for these latter diseases has yet to be demonstrated and there is some immunological evidence that, in scrapie at least (which stands close to the other two), there is progressive physicochemical transformation of cell membranes leading to the emergence of new antigenic determinants which closely resemble (or may indeed be identical with) those which appear in normal ageing tissues both in man and animals.

So far as the general position with regard to transmissibility is concerned, it seems quite likely that the story of poliomyelitis will be repeated in so far as the need for special primates has already yielded to more readily available animals, and there are indications that the agent may survive and increase in titre in tissue culture explants. Whether the agent of scrapie (and kuru and Jakob–Creutzfeldt disease) will turn out to be a 'virus' is an open question. Certainly there is something which can induce consistent changes and itself concomitantly appears in higher concentration. Whether this involves an exception to the Watson–Crick dogma is unclear (Field 1967) but constitutes a fascinating problem in molecular biology.

BIOHAZARDS OF SLOW INFECTIONS

The transmissibility of kuru and Jakob–Creutzfeldt disease from humans to lower animals (albeit under the grossly unusual conditions of experimental inoculation) raises at once the question of infection occurring under ordinary or medical contact conditions. Apart from the bizarre instance of 4 of 7 research workers studying swayback in sheep developing multiple sclerosis (Campbell et al. 1947), there has never been any suggestion of a known slow infection having been contracted in this way. Gajdusek and Gibbs (1973), from their unparalleled experience of kuru and Jakob–Creutzfeldt disease, are of the opinion that 'the epidemiology of the diseases gives no cause for suspicion that the diseases are naturally contagious'. No Caucasian who has come into contact with kuru in the Okapa area of New Guinea has ever developed anything resembling kuru or Jakob–Creutzfeldt disease and the disease remains restricted to the Fore of the area. One case in a non-Fore patient has been reported in a Rabaul newspaper, but this remains unconfirmed (C. J. Gibbs, personal communication). It may be concluded that, under ordinary conditions, kuru is non-infective.

So far as Jakob–Creutzfeldt disease is concerned, infectivity is again very low under ordinary conditions. There is one example of conjugal disease. A 54-year-old neurosurgeon with a clinical diagnosis of papulosis atrophicans maligna (Kohlmeier–Degos disease) was found at post-mortem examination to show changes in the brain consistent with Jakob–Creutzfeldt disease with an additional occasional Cowdry type A inclusion body in oligodendrocytes. From the brain material inoculated into a chimpanzee

and a squirrel monkey both developed typical disease after 26 and
$19\frac{1}{2}$ months' incubation. Whether this really represents an occupa-
tional hazard to neurosurgeons or pathologists is very doubtful,
but clearly it alerts attention. More significant (and indeed
predictable) is the reported development of Jakob–Creutzfeldt
disease in a 55-year-old female recipient of a corneal graft from a
55-year-old man with a two months' history of incoordination,
memory deficit, involuntary movements and myoclonia, and whose
brain at autopsy showed the changes of Jakob–Creutzfeldt disease
(Duffy & Wolf 1974). In effect, introduction of Jakob–Creutzfeldt
material has led to an inadvertent passage experiment in a human.
Other than by introduction of tissues or by ingestion, there would
appear to be very low grade, if any, infectivity. Also, it should be
noted that 'both Jakob–Creutzfeldt and Kuru are transmissible
employing visceral tissues only' (personal communication from
C. J. Gibbs).

'As regards animal caretakers, laboratory technicians, pro-
fessional and non-professional personnel working with human
cases of Kuru and Jakob–Creutzfeldt disease and experimentally
infected animals—we have no evidence even remotely suggesting
infection. In the case of Kuru, this would be more than eighteen
years that non-Fore Negroids and Caucasians have been in close
contact with materials now known to be highly infectious for
animals.' (C. J. Gibbs)

Clearly, contagion is of very low order and the material comes
into the 'low-risk category—meaning that careful handling of the
material in a well trained virus laboratory is acceptable.'

Animal-to-animal contagion is unknown. Despite extensive
experiments in Washington, Louisiana and California, in which
primates have been housed together, no instance of 'contact-
infection' has ever been seen. This applies also to serial passages
of the agents in animal hosts, whereby one might expect to enhance
the virulence. Over the relatively short period kuru and Jakob–
Creutzfeldt infected chimps were in intimate contact at Newcastle
with a normal animal and with one injected with multiple sclerosis,
neither of the latter developed immunological reactions suggestive
of the establishment of an infection.

REFERENCES

Adams, J. M. & Imagawa, D. T. (1962) Measles antibodies in multiple sclerosis. *Proc. Soc. exp. Biol. Med.*, **111**, 562.

Alpers, M. (1965) Epidemiological changes in kuru 1957–1963. In *Slow, Latent and Temperate Virus Infections*, ed. Gajdusek, D. C., Gibbs, C. J. & Alpers, M. NINDB Monograph No. 2. U.S. Department of Health, Education and Welfare.

Asher, D. M. (1971) Russian spring–summer encephalitis. *Proc. XIIIth int. Congr. Pediat.*, 379.

Baker, R. W. R., Thompson, R. H. S. & Zilkha, K. J. (1963) Fatty-acid composition of brain lecithins in multiple sclerosis. *Lancet*, **i**, 26.

Baker, R. W. R., Sanders, H., Thompson, R. H. S. & Zilkha, K. J. (1965) Serum cholesterol linoleate levels in multiple sclerosis. *J. Neurol. Neurosurg. Psychiat.*, **28**, 212.

Barbanti-Brodano, G., Oyanagi, S., Katz, M. & Koprowski, H. (1970) Presence of two different viral agents in brain cells of patients with subacute sclerosing panencephalitis. *Proc. Soc. exp. Biol. Med.*, **134**, 230.

Basnight, M., jun., Rogers, N., Gibbs, C. J., jun. & Gajdusek, D. C. (1970) Characterization of previously undescribed adenoviruses isolated from chimpanzee tissue explants. *Bact. Proc.*, **159**, NIH—91830.

Beck, E., Daniel, P. M., Mathews, W. B., Stevens, D. L., Alpers, M., Asher, D. M., Gajdusek, D. C. & Gibbs, C. J., jun. (1966) Experimental kuru in chimpanzees: a pathological report. *Lancet*, **ii**, 1056.

Bennett, J. H., Rhodes, F. A. & Robson, H. N. (1958) Observations on kuru. I. A possible genetic basis. *Aust. Ann. Med.*, **7**, 269.

Bennett, J. H., Rhodes, F. A. & Robson, H. N. (1959) A possible genetic basis for Kuru. *Am. J. hum. Genet.*, **11**, 169.

Berman, P. H., Giles, J. P. & Krugman, S. (1968) Correlation of measles and subacute sclerosing panencephalitis. *Neurology, Minneap.*, **18**, 91.

Berndt, R. M. (1954) Reaction to contact in the Eastern Highlands of New Guinea. *Oceania*, **24**, 190, 255.

Bonduelle, M., Escourolle, R., Bouygues, P., Lormeau, G., Ribadeau-Dumas, J. R. & Merland, J. J. (1971) Maladie de Creutzfeldt Jakob familiale: observation anatomo-clinique. *Rev. neurol.*, **125**, 197.

Brotherston, J. G., Renwick, C. C., Stamp, J. T., Zlotnik, I. & Pattison, I. H. (1968) Spread of scrapie by contact to goats and sheep. *J. comp. Path.*, **78**, 9.

Buntain, D., Thompson, J. R. & Heath, G. B. S. (1974) Scrapie: observations on a field outbreak. *Vet. Rec.*, **94**, 332.

Burger, D. & Hartshough, G. R. (1965) Transmissible encephalopathy of mink. In *Slow, Latent and Temperate Virus Infections*, ed. Gajdusek, D. C., Gibbs, C. J. & Alpers, M. NINDB Monograph No. 2. U.S. Department of Health, Education and Welfare.

Byington, D. P., Castro, A. E. & Burnstein, T. (1970) Adaptation to hamsters of neurotropic measles virus from subacute sclerosing panencephalitis. *Nature, Lond.*, **225**, 554.

Campbell, A. M. G., Daniel, P., Porter, R. J., Ritchie-Russell, W., Smith, H. V. & Innes, J. R. M. (1947) Disease of the nervous system occurring amongst research workers on swayback in lambs. *Brain*, **70**, 50.

Caspary, E. A., Chambers, M. E. & Field, E. J. (1969) Antibodies to measles antigen, control antigen, and monkey kidney antigen. Studies in patients with multiple sclerosis and other neurological diseases and normal healthy individuals. *Neurology, Minneap.*, **19**, 1038.

Caspary, E. A. & Field, E. J. (1965) An encephalitogenic protein of human origin: some chemical and biological properties. *Ann. N.Y. Acad. Sci.*, **122**, 182.

Caspary, E. A. & Field, E. J. (1970) Sensitization of blood lymphocytes to possible antigens in neurological diseases. *Europ. Neurol.*, **4**, 257.

Caspary, E. A. & Field, E. J. (1971) Specific lymphocyte sensitization in cancer: is there a common antigen in human malignant neoplasia? *Br. med. J.*, **ii**, 613.

Caspary, E. A. & Field, E. J. (1974) Lymphocyte sensitization to basic protein of brain in multiple sclerosis and other neurological diseases. *J. Neurol. Neurosurg. Psychiat.*, **37**, 701.

Chandler, R. L. (1961) Encephalopathy in mice produced by inoculation with scrapiebrain material. *Lancet*, **i**, 1378.

Chandler, R. L. & Fischer, J. (1963) Experimental transmission of scrapie to rats. *Lancet*, **ii**, 1165.

Chelle, P. L. (1942) Un cas de tremblante chez la chèvre. *Bull. Acad. vet. Fr.*, **15**, 294.

Connolly, J. H., Allen, I. V., Hurwitz, L. J. & Millar, J. H. D. (1967) Measles-virus antibody and antigen in subacute sclerosing panencephalitis. *Lancet*, **i**, 542.

Coward, J. E., Harter, D. H. & Morgan, C. (1970) Electron-microscopic observations of visna virus-infected cell cultures. *Virology*, **40**, 1030.

Davison, C. & Rabiner, A. M. (1940) Spastic pseudosclerosis. *Archs Neurol. Psychiat.*, **44**, 578.

Dick, G. W. A., McAlister, J. J., McKeown, F. & Campbell, A. M. G. (1965) Multiple sclerosis and scrapie. *J. Neurol. Neurosurg. Psychiat.*, **28**, 560.

Dickinson, A. G., Stamp, J. T. & Renwick, C. C. (1974) Maternal and lateral spread of scrapie in sheep. *J. comp. Path.*, **84**, 19.

Duffy, P. & Wolf, J. (1974) Possible person-to-person transmission of Creutzfeldt–Jakob disease. *New Engl. J. Med.*, **134**, 692.

Eckroade, R. J., Zu Rhein, G. M., Marsh, R. F. & Hanson, R. P. (1969) Transmissible mink encephalopathy: experimental transmission to the squirrel monkey. *Science, N.Y.*, **169**, 1088.

Field, E. J. (1966) Transmission experiments with multiple sclerosis: an interim report. *Br. med. J.*, **ii**, 564.

Field, E. J. (1967a) Invasion of the nervous system by scrapie agent. *Br. J. exp. Path.*, **48**, 662.

Field, E. J. (1967b) Spread of scrapie agent by the blood stream. *Vet. Rec.*, **81**, 495.

Field, E. J. (1967c) The significance of astroglial hypertrophy in scrapie, Kuru, multiple sclerosis and old age, together with a note on the possible nature of the scrapie agent. *Dt. Z. NervHeilk.*, **192**, 265.

Field, E. J. (1969) Slow virus infections of the nervous system. *Int. Rev. exp. Path.*, **8**, 129.

Field, E. J. (1973) Rôle of viral infections and auto-immunity in aetiology and pathogenesis of multiple sclerosis. *Lancet*, **i**, 295.

Field, E. J. & Caspary, E. A. (1970) Lymphocyte sensitization: an *in vitro* test for cancer? *Lancet*, **ii**, 1337.

Field, E. J. & Caspary, E. A. (1971) Demonstration of sensitized lymphocytes in blood. *J. clin. Path.*, **24**, 179.

Field, E. J., Caspary, E. A., Shenton, B. K. & Madgwick, H. (1973) Lymphocyte sensitization after exposure to measles and influenza: possible relevance to pathogenesis of multiple sclerosis. *J. Neurol. Sci.*, **19**, 179.

Field, E. J. & Joyce, G. (1970) Evidence against transmission of scrapie by animal house fomites. *Nature, Lond.*, **226**, 791.

Field, E. J., Joyce, G. & Keith, A. (1969) Failure of interferon to modify scrapie in the mouse. *J. gen. Virol.*, **5**, 149.

Field, E. J. & McDermott, J. R. (1973) Measles and multiple sclerosis. *Lancet*, **i**, 376.

Field, E. J. & Shenton, B. K. (1972) Rapid diagnosis of scrapie in the mouse. *Nature, Lond.*, **240**, 104.

Field, E. J. & Shenton, B. K. (1973a) Immunological reactions in scrapie: the basis of a rapid titration method. *Path. Biol.*, **21**, 1051.

Field, E. J. & Shenton, B. K. (1973b) Retardation of ageing in mice by implants of thymus tissue. *IRCS*, (73–6), 5–10–3.

Field, E. J. & Shenton, B. K. (1973c) Emergence of new antigens in ageing tissues. *Gerontologia*, **19**, 211.

Field, E. J. & Shenton, B. K. (1973d) Thymectomy and immunological ageing in mice; precocious emergence of scrapie-like antigen. *Gerontologia*, **19**, 203.

Field, E. J. & Shenton, B. K. (1973e) Altered response to scrapie tissue in neurological disease: possible evidence for an antigen associated with reactive astrocytes. *Brain*, **96**, 629.

Field, E. J. & Shenton, B. K. (1974a) A rapid immunologic test for scrapie in sheep. *Am. J. vet. Res.*, **35**, 393.

Field, E. J. & Shenton, B. K. (1974b) Cellular sensitization in slow infections of the nervous system: comparison of Kuru, Jakob–Creutzfeldt disease and multiple sclerosis. In the press.

Field, E. J., Shenton, B. K. & Joyce, G. (1974a) Specific laboratory test for diagnosis of multiple sclerosis. *Br. med. J.*, **i**, 412.

Field, E. J., Shenton, B. K., Joyce, G. & Buntain, D. (1974b) Multiple sclerosis and scrapie. *IRCS*, **2**, 1041.

Field, E. J. & Windsor, G. D. (1966) Cultural characters of scrapie mouse brain. *Res. vet. Sci.*, **6**, 160.

Fischer, A. & Fischer, J. L. (1960) Aetiology of kuru. *Lancet*, **i**, 1417.

Fischer, A. & Fischer, J. L. (1963) Culture and epidemiology: a theoretical investigation of kuru. *J. Hlth Hum. Behav.*, **2**, 16.

Friede, R. L. & De Jong, R. N. (1964) Neuronal enzymatic failure in Creutzfeldt–Jakob disease (a familial study). *Archs Neurol., Chicago,* **10**, 181.

Gajdusek, D. C. (1971) Slow virus diseases of the central nervous system. *Am. J. clin. Path.*, **56**, 320.

Gajdusek, D. C. & Gibbs, C. J., jun. (1964) Attempts to demonstrate a transmissible agent in Kuru, amyotrophic lateral sclerosis and other subacute and chronic nervous system degenerations of man. *Nature, Lond.*, **204**, 257.

Gajdusek, D. C. & Gibbs, C. J., jun. (1971) Transmission of the spongiform encephalopathies of man (Kuru and Creutzfeldt–Jakob disease) to New World monkeys. *Nature, Lond.*, **230**, 588.

Gajdusek, D. C. & Gibbs, C. J., jun. (1972) Transmission of Kuru from man to rhesus monkey (*Macaca mulatta*) 8½ years after inoculation. *Nature, Lond.*, **240**, 351.

Gajdusek, D. C. & Gibbs, C. J., jun. (1973) Subacute and chronic diseases caused by atypical infections with unconventional viruses in aberrant hosts. *Perspect. Virol.*, **8**, 279.

Gajdusek, D. C., Gibbs, C. J., jun. & Alpers, M. (1965) *Slow, Latent and Temperate Virus Infections*, NINDB Monograph No. 2. U.S. Department of Health, Education and Welfare.

Gajdusek, D. C., Gibbs, C. J., jun. & Alpers, M. (1966) Experimental transmission of a Kuru-like syndrome to chimpanzees. *Nature, Lond.*, **209**, 794.

Gajdusek, D. C., Gibbs, C. J., jun., Asher, D. & David, E. (1968) Transmission of experimental Kuru to the spider monkey (*Ateles geoffroyi*). *Science, N.Y.*, **162**, 693.

Gajdusek, D. C., Gibbs, C. J., jun., Earle, K., Dammin, C. J., Schoene, W. C. & Tyler, H. R. (1975) Transmission of subacute spongiform encephalopathy to the chimpanzee and squirrel monkey from a patient with papulosis atrophicans maligna (Kohlmeier-Degos disease). In the press.

Gajdusek, D. C., Gibbs, C. J., jun., Rogers, N. G., Basnight, M. & Hooks, J. (1972) Persistence of viruses of Kuru and Creutzfeldt–Jakob disease in tissue cultures of brain cells. *Nature, Lond.*, **235**, 104.

Gajdusek, D. C. & Zigas, V. (1957) Degenerative disease of the central nervous system in New Guinea. The endemic occurrence of Kuru in the native population. *New Engl. J. Med.*, **257**, 974.

Gardner, A. C. (1965) Gel diffusion reactions to tissue and sera from scrapie affected animals. *Res. vet. Sci.*, **7**, 190.

Gibbs, C. J. & Gajdusek, D. C. (1971) Transmission and characterization of the agents of spongiform virus encephalopathies: Kuru, Creutzfeldt–Jakob disease, scrapie and mink encephalopathy. In *Immunological Disorders of the Nervous System*, ed. Rowland, L. P. *Res. nerv. ment. Dis.*, **49**, 383.

Gibbs, C. J., jun., Gajdusek, D. C., Asher, D. M., Alpers, M. P., Beck, E., Daniel, P. M. & Mathews, W. B. (1968) Creutzfeldt–Jakob disease (subacute spongiform encephalopathy): transmission to the chimpanzee. *Science, N.Y.*, **161**, 388.

Gordon, W. S. (1966) *Report of the Scrapie Seminar*, p. 19. Washington D.C.: U.S. Department of Agriculture.

Gresser, I. & Pattison, I. H. (1968) An attempt to modify scrapie in mice by the administration of interferon. *J. gen. Virol.*, **3**, 295.

Gustaffson, D. P. & Kanitz, C. L. (1965) Evidence of the presence of scrapie in cell cultures of brain. In *Slow, Latent and Temperate Virus Infections*, ed. Gajdusek, D. C., Gibbs, C. J., jun. & Alpers, M. NINDB Monograph No. 2. U.S. Department of Health, Education and Welfare.

Hadlow, W. J. (1959) Scrapie and kuru. *Lancet*, **ii**, 289.

Haig, D. A. & Clarke, M. C. (1971) Culture of scrapie agent. *Nature, Lond.*, **234**, 106.

Haig, D. A. & Pattison, I. H. (1967) *In vitro* growth of pieces of brain from scrapie affected mice. *J. Path. Bact.*, **93**, 724.

Harter, D. H. (1969) Observations on the plaque assay of visna virus. *J. gen. Virol.*, **5**, 157.

Harter, D. H., Hsu, K. C. & Rose, H. M. (1968) Multiplication of visna virus in bovine and porcine cell lines. *Proc. Soc. exp. Biol. Med.*, **129**, 295.

Henson, T. E., Brody, J. A., Sever, J. L., Dyken, M. L. & Cannon, J. (1970) Measles antibody titres in multiple sclerosis, siblings and controls. *J. Am. med. Ass.*, **211**, 1185.

Horta-Barbosa, L., Sever, J. L., Ley, A., Krebs, H. M. & Gilkeson, M. R. (1970) Progressive increase in cerebrospinal fluid measles antibody levels in subacute sclerosing panencephalitis. *Fedn Proc. Fedn Am. Socs exp. Biol.*, **29**, 436.

Hourrigan, J. L., Klingsporn, A. L., McDaniel, H. & Riemenschneider, M. N. (1969) Natural scrapie in a goat. *J. Am. vet. Med. Ass.*, **154**, 538.

Jellinger, K. & Seitelberger, F. (1972) Konjugale Form der subakuten spongiöser Enzephalopathie. *Wien. klin. Wschr.*, **84**, 245.

Johnson, R. T. (1970) Subacute sclerosing panencephalitis. Editorial. *J. infect. Dis.*, **121**, 227.

Just, M., Rieder, H. P. & Ritzel, G. (1967) Measles antibody in serum of multiple sclerosis patients. *Klin. Wschr.*, **45**, 707.

Katz, M., Rorke, L. B., Masland, W. S., Barbanti-Brodano, G. & Koprowski, H. (1970) Subacute sclerosing panencephalitis: isolation of a virus encephalitogenic for ferrets. *J. infect. Dis.*, **121**, 188.

Latz, M., Rorke, L. B., Masland, W. C., Koprowski, H. & Tucker, S. H. (1968) Transmission of an encephalitogenic agent from brains of patients with subacute sclerosing panencephalitis to ferrets. *New Engl. J. Med.*, **279**, 793.

Kim, C. S., Kriewalt, F. H., Magino, N. & Kalter, S. S. (1970) Subacute sclerosing panencephalitis-like syndrome in the adult baboon (*Papro* sp.). *J. Am. vet. med. Ass.*, **157**, 730.

Kirschbaum, W. R. (1968) *Jakob-Creutzfeldt Disease*. New York: Elsevier.

Klatzo, I., Gajdusek, D. C. & Zigas, V. (1959) Pathology of Kuru. *Lab. Invest.*, **8,** 799.

Klippel, J. H., Decker, J. L., Grimley, P. M., Evans, A. S. & Rothfield, N. F. (1973) Epstein–Barr virus antibody and lymphocyte tubulo-reticular structures in systemic lupus erythematosus. *Lancet*, **ii,** 1057.

Koprowski, H., Barbanto-Brodano, G. & Katz, M. (1970) Interaction between papova-like virus and paramyxovirus in human brain cells: a hypothesis. *Nature, Lond.*, **225,** 1045.

Laitinen, O. & Vaheri, A. (1974) Very high measles and rubella virus antibody titres associated with hepatitis, systemic lupus erythematosus and infectious mononucleosis. *Lancet*, **i,** 194.

Lehrich, J. R., Katz, M., Rorke, L. B., Barbanti-Brodano, G. & Koprowski, H. (1970) Subacute sclerosing panencephalitis. Encephalitis produced in hamsters by viral agents isolated from human brain cells. *Archs Neurol., Chicago*, **23,** 97.

McAlpine, D., Lumsden, C. E. & Acheson, E. D. (1972) *Multiple Sclerosis: A Reappraisal*, 2nd ed. Edinburgh and London: Churchill Livingstone.

McDermott, J., Field, E. J. & Caspary, E. A. (1974) Relation of measles virus to encephalitogenic factor with reference to the aetiopatho-genesis of multiple sclerosis. *J. Neurol. Neurosurg. Psychiat.*, **37,** 282.

Mackay, J. M. K. & Smith, W. (1961) A case of scrapie in an uninoculated goat—a natural occurrence or a contact infection? *Vet. Rec.*, **73,** 394.

Mackay, R. P. & Myrianthopoulos, N. C. (1966) Multiple sclerosis in twins and their relations. *Archs Neurol., Chicago*, **15,** 449.

Marsh, R. F., Burger, D., Eckroade, R. J., Zu Rhein, G. M. & Hanson, R. P. (1969) A preliminary report on the experimental host range of the transmissible mink encephalopathy agent. *J. infect. Dis.*, **120,** 713.

Mertin, J., Shenton, B. K. & Field, E. J. (1973) Lymphocyte reactivity in relation to unsaturated fatty acids in blood; with special reference to multiple sclerosis. *Br. med. J.*, **ii,** 777.

Ter Meulen, V., Enders-Ruckle, G., Müller, D. & Joppich, G. (1969) Immunohistological microscopical and neurochemical studies on encephalitides. III. subacute progressive panencephalitis. Virological and immunohistological studies. *Acta neuropath.*, **12,** 244.

Ter Meulen, V., Katz, M. & Oyanagi, S. (1970) Differences in intracellular antigen distribution between SSPE (subacute sclerosing panencephalitis) viruses and measles viruses. *Fedn Proc. Fedn Am. Socs exp. Biol.*, **29,** 436.

Ter Meulen, V., Koprowski, H., Iwasaki, Y., Käckel, Y. M. & Müller. D. (1972) Fusion of cultured multiple sclerosis brain cells with indicator cells: presence of nucleocapsids and virions and isolation of para-influenza type virus. *Lancet*, **ii,** 1.

Millar, J. H. D., Zilkha, K. J., Langman, M. J. S., Payling-Wright, H., Smith, A. D., Belin, J. & Thompson, R. H. S. (1973) Double blind trial of linoleate supplementation of the diet in multiple sclerosis. *Br. med. J.*, **i,** 765.

Narang, H. K. & Field, E. J. (1973) Paramyxovirus-like tubules in multiple sclerosis biopsy material. *Acta neuropath.*, **25**, 281.

Narang, H. K., Shenton, B. K., Giorgi, P. P. & Field, E. J. (1972) Scrapie agent and neurones. *Nature, Lond.*, **240**, 105.

Niedermeyer, E., Gibbs, C. J., jun., Marsh, R. & Gajdusek, D. C. (1972) EEG studies in subacute and degenerative neurological diseases experimentally produced in ferrets and chimpanzees. *Electroenceph. clin. Neurophysiol.*, **33**, 351.

Norton, W. R. (1969) Electron microscopic observations of lymphocytes in systemic lupus erythematosus. *J. Lab. clin. Med.*, **74**, 369.

Palsson, P. A., Pattison, I. H. & Field, E. J. (1965) Transmission experiments with multiple sclerosis. In *Slow, Latent and Temperate Virus Infections*, ed. Gajdusek, D. C., Gibbs, C. J., jun. & Alpers, M. NINDB Monograph No. 2. U.S. Department of Health, Education and Welfare.

Parry, H. B. (1962) Scrapie: a transmissible hereditary disease of sheep. *Heredity*, **17**, 75.

Parry, H. B. (1966) *Report of the Scrapie Seminar*, p. 125. Washington D.C.: U.S. Department of Agriculture.

Pattison, I. H. (1964) The spread of scrapie by contact between affected and healthy sheep, goats or mice. *Vet. Rec.*, **76**, 333.

Pattison, I. H., Gordon, W. S. & Millson, G. C. (1959) Experimental production of scrapie in goats. *J. comp. Path.*, **69**, 300.

Pattison, I. H., Hoare, M. N., Jebbett, J. N. & Watson, W. A. (1972) Spread of scrapie to sheep and goats by oral dosing with foetal membranes from scrapie-affected sheep. *Vet. Rec.*, **90**, 465.

Pattison, I. H. & Jebbett, J. N. (1971) Clinical and histological observations on cuprizone toxicity and scrapie in mice. *Res. vet. Sci.*, **12**, 378.

Pattison, I. H. & Millson, G. C. (1961) Experimental transmission of scrapie to goats and sheep by the oral route. *J. comp. Path. Ther.*, **71**, 171.

Payne, F. E. (1971) Measles virus and subacute sclerosing panencephalitis. *Perspect. Virol.*, **7**.

Périer, O., Thiry, L., Vanderhaeghen, J. J. & Pelc, S. (1968) Attempts at experimental transmission and electron microscopic observations in subacute sclerosing panencephalitis. *Neurology, Minneap.*, **18**, 138.

Prineas, J. (1972) Paramyxovirus-like particles associated with acute demyelination in chronic relapsing multiple sclerosis. *Science, N.Y.*, **178**, 760.

Ressang, A. A., Stam, F. C. & De Boer, G. F. (1966) A meningoleukencephalomyelitis resembling visna in Dutch zwoeger sheep. *Path. vet.*, **3**, 401.

Ross, C. A. C., Lenman, J. A. & Rutter, C. (1965) Infective agents and multiple sclerosis. *Br. med. J.*, **i**, 226.

Schaltenbrand, G., Trostdorf, E., Henn, R. & Orthner, H. (1968) Kuruähnliche sklerosierende Panencephalomyelitis in Europa. *Dt. Z. NervHeilk.*, **193**, 158.

Schapira, K., Poskanzer, D. C. & Miller, H. G. (1963) Familial and conjugal multiple sclerosis. *Brain*, **86**, 315.

Sever, J. L. & Kurtzke, J. F. (1969) Delayed dermal hypersensitivity to measles and mumps antigens among multiple sclerosis and control patients. *Neurology, Minneap.*, **19**, 113.

Shenton, B. K., Buntain, D., Field, E. J. & Joyce, G. (1975) Incubation of scrapie under natural conditions; immunological and clinical observations. In the press.

Sigurdsson, B. (1954) Observations on three slow infections of sheep. *Br. vet. J.*, **110**, 255, 307, 341.

Sigurdsson, B., Palsson, P. A. & Grimsson, H. (1957) Visna; a demyelinating transmissible disease of sheep. *J. Neuropath. exp. Neurol.*, **16**, 389.

Stamp, J. T. (1962) Scrapie: a transmissible disease of sheep. *Vet. Rec.*, **74**, 357.

Sutherland, J. M. & Wilson, D. R. (1951) Disseminated sclerosis in man and experimentation with sheep. *Glasg. med. J.*, **32**, 302.

Thompson, R. H. S. (1966) A biochemical approach to the problem of multiple sclerosis. *Proc. R. Soc. Med.*, **59**, 269.

Thormar, H. (1967) Cell-virus interactions in tissue cultures infected with visna and maedi viruses. *Curr. Topics Microbiol. Immunol.*, **40**, 22.

Thormar, H. (1971) Slow infections of the central nervous system. *Z. Neurol.*, **199**, 151.

Thormar, H. & Palsson, P. A. (1967) Visna and maedi—two slow infections of sheep and their etiological aspects. *Perspect. Virol.*, **5**, 291.

Turnell, R. W., Clarke, L. H. & Burton, A. F. (1973) Studies on the mechanism of cortico-steroid induced lymphocytolysis. *Cancer Res.*, **33**, 203.

Williams, F. E. (1923) *Territ. Papua anthrop. Rep.* Port Moresby, **73**, 78.

Zlotnik, I. (1963) Experimental transmission of scrapie to golden hamsters. *Lancet*, **ii**, 1072.

Zu Rhein, G. M. (1969a) Association of papova-virions with a human demyelinating disease (progressive multifocal leukoencephalopathy). *Progr. med. Virol.*, **11**, 185.

Zu Rhein, G. M. (1969b) Discussion. Pathogenesis and aetiology of demyelinating diseases. *Int. Arch. Allergy*, **36**, 604.

12

The Future

G. W. A. DICK

In the future we shall require:

1. Better and more rapid laboratory methods of diagnosis by isolation or serology.
2. Better epidemiology.
3. A better understanding of the pathogenesis of viruses infecting the CNS.

Methods to provide more rapid diagnosis by fluorescent and other techniques have not so far met with success in all hands, but there is a great need for such methods and this is particularly so when more suitable antiviral substances are developed.

Considerable progress has been made by immunologists in measuring the different classes of antibody, but there is now some doubt whether the demonstration of specific IgM in serum or CSF is necessarily indicative of a very recent virus infection. If IgM is found in the CSF or serum, could this not be merely dependent on the life span of the cells synthesizing it? It does not necessarily seem to mean the continuing presence (or recent presence) of the antigen which stimulated it.

I think in the future we should study not just 'antibody' but the levels of IgG and IgM in the sera and CSF of all unexplained neurological diseases.

As we all know so well, in many cases of presumed viral infections of the CNS, no virus is ever recovered. We should be making more efforts to use methods of co-cultivation which are so successful in the recovery of measles virus in SSPE and utilizing techniques involving 'helper' viruses.

As far as epidemiology is concerned, many seem to have forgotten that only by asking 'when', 'where' and 'amongst whom' does a disease occur, can we ask 'why'. Good notifications are essential for accurate epidemiological inferences and it is most depressing how poor the notifications of encephalitis generally are. Only when we have complete data with an accurate diagnosis and the 'time', 'place' and 'person' of the disease, can we begin to understand its natural history, to define the extent of the problem and to consider methods for its control or prevention.

With many virus diseases of the CNS, we often hear only about the tip of the iceberg. I do not believe that all cases of 'activation' of measles virus in the CNS lead to SSPE and there may be many demented children who have not progressed to the classical picture of SSPE which is seen in children's hospitals. Similarly, there must be a spectrum of CNS infections caused by herpes simplex virus. Is anyone diagnosing mild cases? All CNS infections with herpes simplex virus cannot lead to severe necrotizing encephalitis. It is important to try to identify the less severe infections, for they might be more readily susceptible to therapy with idoxuridine or cytosine arabinoside.

As far as pathogenesis is concerned, it has become more clear nowadays that the resultant pathology in CNS infections is in part due to the immune response to the viral antigens. The immune response is, of course, usually beneficial, but if it is harmful could it be modified? I am no immunologist, but it seems that as far as the humoral response is concerned, if the antibody does not 'remove' the antigen from the CNS, then there may be an Arthus type of reaction and immune complexes may give rise to chronic inflammatory changes and degenerative disease. It has been said by some that antibody may prevent cell recognition and inhibit cell mediated immunity (CMI). Furthermore, the importance of humoral antibody on the outcome of an infection is appreciated, when it is remembered that the attachment of antibody to the surface of infected cells may accelerate phagocytosis and with complement and virus may cause cell destruction. Should we study this problem in animal models in more detail?

It is of some interest that in Japanese B encephalitis and in Aleutian mink disease, passive immunization may intensify the lesions. On the other hand, in some neurotropic virus infections, passive immunization may delay the onset of paralysis but in the long run such paralysis is intensified. Would immune suppression influence the outcome? Obviously, this requires further study.

It appears that some viruses, e.g. lymphocytic choriomeningitis, can selectively depress T cells, and measles and rubella virus are said to be able to inhibit blast formation. It seems sensible to study the effect of viruses on B and T cells: if the T cells are inadequate then the virus is not cleared and the B cells may then proliferate; this may not only result in the synthesis of antiviral antibody but may also give rise to autoimmune reactions.

Would immunosuppression have any effect in those diseases which seem to involve CMI and humoral immunity in pathogenesis, e.g. SSPE? It would seem worth trying its effect.

In some virus infections in animals, it has been shown that cyclophosphamide greatly reduces the inflammatory lesions. It is said that it exerts this influence by inhibiting or destroying sensitized lymphocytes (which presumably affect both CMI and humoral antibody synthesis). We have been told, earlier, that the CNS lesions in cyclophosphamide treated primates looks like the spongy encephalopathy of kuru, scrapie, Jakob–Creutzfeldt disease and mink encephalopathy. Although none of the agents of these diseases produce any demonstrable antibodies, does anyone know what levels of immunoglobulins are found in the CSF in the various species infected with these agents?

Returning to the question of immunosuppression. Have we any useful repeatable experimental data on the effect of anti-lymphocytic serum on degenerative conditions of the CNS? As far as I can see, the results of using anti-lymphocytic serum are very inconclusive. Presumably, ALS influences CMI and also humoral antibody production and indeed from the investigations

I have read, the effect of anti-lymphocytic serum seems to be influenced by all sorts of things, even PK!

Recently, many people have got on to the bandwagon of the genetic control of susceptibility and searches are being made to see if there is an association between HLA, phenotype and susceptibility. It has been known for many years that there were racial and familial susceptibilities to many diseases, e.g. it is known that from time to time, two cases of poliomyelitis occur in one family and that occasionally there seems to be a familial factor in multiple sclerosis. The recent observations that LD7A histocompatibility antigens are more frequent in multiple sclerosis patients than in controls may not add much to our knowledge of the pathogenesis of the disease, unless these antigens are associated with genes which influence the host response and which could be artificially altered.

Much of the new information on multiple sclerosis suggests that the disease is multifactorial and that at least one of the responsible antigens may be a measles virus of a more incomplete character than the incomplete virus which causes SSPE.

I know little about the induction of new antigens on the cell surfaces by viruses infecting the CNS, but the induction of such new antigens on cell surfaces may react with antibody or sensitized lymphocytes and produce destruction of cells.

For completion, it might be mentioned that some viruses invade the mononuclear phagocytic system (e.g. SSPE and EB virus) and this may have a profound effect on the immune mechanism of the host.

The one disease we should all like to understand is multiple sclerosis, but perhaps when we discover that it has a multifactorial aetiology it may not be very easy to prevent it: if it is simple anergy to measles and a selective CMI deficiency, then perhaps this deficiency might be mended or the anergy reversed under some conditions by transfer factor.

What about other degenerative disease? What about CNS diseases with no obvious pathology such as schizophrenia? It is said that a disproportional number of schizophrenics are born in the first quarter of the year. Is there a viral aetiology?

In all investigations, both clinical and non-clinical, we must always remember the scientific method and never forget that *libenter homines in quod volunt credunt* (man prefers to believe what he prefers to be true).

Index

Index